Table of Contents.

Introduction to Dysphagia	4
Warning Signs of Dysphagia	9
The Dysphagia Care Team	10
Special Considerations During Mealtime	13
General Guidelines for Puree Diets	14
Thickened Liquids	19
Preparation Suggestions for Puree Diets	27
Puree Recipe Principles	30
Preserving Nutrients in Puree Food Preparation	30
Kitchen Equipment and Processing Tips	31
General Food Safety	32
Proper Cooking Temperatures	33
Increasing Calories and Protein in Puree Meals	34
What are healthy food choices?	36
How much food to serve?	44
Sample Meal Plans with Calorie Levels	44
Common Portion Sizes for Puree Foods	48
Recipes	49
Beverages	49
Breads	56
Desserts	60
Entrees	65
Entrees Beef	67
Entrees Chicken	71
Entrees Pork	86
Entrees Seafood	92
Entrée Turkey	101
Fruits	106
Salad Dressing	107
Sauces	119
Soups	136
Starch Side Dishes	145
Vegetables	151
Vegetable Salads	153
Vegetable Smoothies	155

Introduction to Dysphasia:

People with dysphagia have difficulty swallowing and may experience pain while swallowing. Some people may be unable to swallow or may have trouble swallowing liquids, foods, or saliva. Eating then can become a challenge. Often, dysphasia makes it difficult to take in enough calories and fluids to nourish the body.

Swallowing is a complex process. Some fifty pairs of muscles and many nerves are involved in the movement of from the mouth to the stomach. This happens in four stages. The first phase is also known as the "anticipatory phase" is called the oral preparatory stage. The oral preparatory phase occurs before the food ever reaches the mouth. The senses are stimulated by the appearance and aroma of food. These sensations affect the willingness to eat or accept food. For some people the impaired sensation of smell or sight or with nausea food may not seem appealing. The desire to eat foods may become a daily task.

The second phase, is the normal swallow or voluntary action of moving the food (or bolus) to the back of the into the mouth (pharynx) to be swallowed. This is called the oral phase. In the oral phase, the tongue moves the food around in the mouth for chewing. Chewing makes the food the right size to swallow and helps mix the food with saliva. Saliva softens and moistens the food to make swallowing easier. Food temperature, textures, and moisture may affect the ease or difficulty of the oral phase of swallowing. Individuals with dysphasia may have lost the ability to perform this simple task or the task is impaired. During this second stage, the tongue collects the prepared food or liquid, making it ready for swallowing. The collection of food is called a bolus.

The third stage phase is called the pharyngeal phase. In a normal swallow, this phase is an involuntary action that begins when the bolus of food reaches the back of the throat and the swallow response is then triggered. This response begins when the tongue pushes the food or liquid to the back of the mouth, which triggers a swallowing reflex that passes the food through the pharynx (the canal that connects the mouth with the esophagus). During this stage, the larynx (voice box) closes tightly and breathing stops to prevent food or liquid from entering the lungs. In the normal swallow this actions takes less than one second. Temperature, taste and texture of the food can all affect the response speed of the swallow. The viscosity (thickness) of liquids can affect the speed at which liquids moves in the throat. Thin liquids usually move faster than thick liquids and may be harder to control for some individuals. People with dysphasia may have a delayed, incomplete or absent swallow response. Normally the larynx lifts and closes to protect the airway. If the sequences do not occur completely or is mistimed, the consumer is at risk for aspiration. In an abnormal swallow, food or fluid may become trapped in the pharynx (the area of the throat just behind the mouth). The larynx (voice box) may not properly lift or close as to prevent from going into the airway. If the larynx is not working properly food may go into the airway causing choking or difficulty breathing.

The final is the esophageal phase is also an involuntary phase in the normal swallow. In this stage begins when food or liquid enters the esophagus, the canal that carries food and liquid to the stomach. This passage through the esophagus usually occurs in about 3-9 seconds, depending on the texture or consistency of the food.

Dysphasia occurs when there is a problem with any part of the swallowing process. Weak tongue or cheek muscles may make it hard to move food around in the mouth for chewing. Food pieces that are too large for swallowing may enter the throat and block the passage of air.

Other problems include not being able to start the swallowing reflex (a stimulus that allows food and liquids to move safely through the pharynx) because of a stroke or other nervous system disorder. People with these kinds of problems are unable to begin the muscle movements that allow food to move from the mouth to the stomach. Another difficulty can occur when weak throat muscles cannot move all the food toward the stomach. Bits of food can fall or be pulled into the windpipe (trachea), which may result in lung infection or aspiration pneumonia.

Sometimes, when foods or liquids enter the windpipe of a person who has dysphasia, coughing or throat clearing cannot remove it. Food or liquid that stays in the windpipe may enter the lungs and create a chance for harmful bacteria to grow. A serious infection (aspiration pneumonia) can result.

Swallowing disorders may also include the development of a pocket outside the esophagus caused by weakness in the esophageal wall. This abnormal pocket traps some food being swallowed. While lying down or sleeping, a person with this problem may draw undigested food into the pharynx. The esophagus may be too narrow, causing food to stick. This food may prevent other food or even liquids from entering the stomach.

Dysphasia has many causes. Any condition that weakens or damages the muscles and nerves used for swallowing may cause dysphasia. For example, people with diseases of the nervous system, such as cerebral palsy or Parkinson's disease, often have problems swallowing. Additionally, stroke or head injury may affect the coordination of the swallowing muscles or limit sensation in the mouth and throat. An infection or irritation can cause narrowing of the esophagus. People born with abnormalities of the swallowing mechanism may not be able to swallow normally. Infants who are born with a hole in the roof of the mouth (cleft palate) are unable to suck properly, which complicates nursing and drinking from a regular baby bottle.

In addition, cancer of the head, neck, or esophagus may cause swallowing problems. Sometimes the treatment for these types of cancers can cause dysphasia. Injuries of the head, neck, and chest may also create swallowing problems.

Dysphasia is not a disease but a disruption of a normal process. Dysphasia can lead to silent aspiration. Silent aspiration occurs when food or fluid enters the lungs with no immediate physical signs of a problem. Silent aspiration can occur before, during or after the swallow.
Aspiration pneumonia is the fifth leading cause of death in people over 60 years of age and third leading cause of death in people over 80.

Dysphasia can be serious. Someone who cannot swallow well may not be able to eat enough of the right foods to stay healthy or maintain an ideal weight. Increasing calories, by fortifying foods with nutrient dense high calorie foods may assist in maintaining a healthy weight. If a person with dysphagia has difficulty maintaining a healthy weight by eating foods orally, alternate methods of feeding may need to be considered. A feeding tube can provide additional nutrients to maintain good health. A feeding tube does NOT mean all oral feeding must be discontinued. Foods can still be enjoyed as tolerated if the person is not aspirating foods and just has difficulty maintaining adequate nourishment for weight maintenance. A feeding tube can be used in conjunction with eating orally too. For optional nutrition, it is usually best to avoid a progressive weight loss and provide adequate nourishment. Weekly monitoring of weight is recommended for individuals with dysphagia. A progressive weight loss or gain should be reported to the medical doctor. When considering a feeding tube for nourishment, a medical doctor and registered dietitian nutritionist should be consulted.

Preparing Puree Meals

This publication was developed for and under the direction and supervision of the Jacqueline Larson M.S., R.D.N and Associates. All rights under federal copyright laws are held by Jacqueline Larson M.S. R.D.N. and Associates.

All parts of this publication may not be reproduced in any form of printed or visual medium. Any reproduction of this publication may not be sold for profit or reproduction costs without the exclusive permission of Jacqueline Larson M.S., R.D.N and Associates. Any reproduction of this manual in whole or part, shall acknowledge Jacqueline Larson M.S., R.D.N. and Associates in writing.

PREFACE

Dysphagia is a growing problem in the United States. Dysphagia means difficulty with chewing or swallowing food and/ or liquid. Dysphagia can be serious. Someone who cannot swallow or chew well may not be able to eat enough of the right foods to stay healthy or maintain an ideal weight

With the aging population, care providers are may need to modify the meals to facilitate an easier method for swallowing. Although there are different levels of chewing and swallowing difficulty, this book focuses on the preparation of puree meals. Chewing and swallowing is a very complex process. Some fifty pairs of muscles and many nerves work to move food from the mouth to the stomach. Everyone's nutritional and diet modification needs are different. Individuals with chewing and swallowing difficulty are at greater risk for complications like aspiration pneumonia or choking.

DISCLAIMER

The information provided here is as up to date, accurate and as practical as possible in a field that moving very quickly and is full of controversy. Any preparations in this cookbook should be discussed with and managed by your medical physician. The implementation should be supervised by a registered dietitian/nutritionist. It is highly recommended individuals with chewing and/or swallowing difficulties consult with a qualified Speech and Language Pathologist and/or qualified Occupational Therapeutists. Great effort has been taken to assure the accuracy of this book, however, we know that errors do occur and caution should be used when feeding or preparing meals of individuals with special needs. The author and publisher disclaim any responsibility for any adverse consequences resulting from the use of this book.

Undetected or untreated dysphasia can lead to many serious health problems including:

Aspiration

Choking

Dehydration

Malnutrition

Potential for depression due to inability to consume desirable foods and fluids

People who are likely to develop dysphasia include those who have:

- Poor dentition or poor mouth care
- Cerebral vascular accident or stroke (CVA)
- Neuromuscular diseases such as Parkinson's disease, Huntington Chorea, or Multiple Sclerosis
- Cerebral Palsy
- Cancer of the head, neck or esophagus
- Radiation treatment to the head or neck area
- Trauma to the esophagus, tongue, larynx or pharynx
- Repeated pneumonias
- Dementia especially at the end stage of Alzheimer's disease
- Head injury or spinal injury
- People who are on medications that cause sedation, impaired cognition or decrease production of salvia

The first step in treatment is to make the proper diagnosis. This involves a medical history and various tests to find the cause of the dysphagia. Often a team approach to treatment is needed. Several types of health care providers -- physicians, registered dietitian, psychologist, speech pathologist, occupational therapist -- work together to develop the best program.

An important part of the treatment is helping the patient get adequate nutrition, while protecting against complications such as pneumonia from food or liquid getting into the lungs. This requires a specialized diet. There are different diet levels from puréed, ground, chopped and regular. (The terminology may vary.)
In order to create a better framework for texture modified diets internationally, the International Dysphagia Diet Standardisation Initiative (IDDSI) was founded in 2013. The goal of the group is to standardize the way of naming and describing texture modified foods and thickened liquids for people with dysphagia. Standardization of dysphagia diets is to promote patient safety and to facilitate evolution of the field to deliver better treatment outcomes.
Eight levels of the dysphagia diets exist. Liquids are measured from levels 0-4 and Foods are measured 3-7. Level 4 is pureed. Foods and liquids can fit into the puree level. Foods need in the puree level need to be smooth, cohesive, should not be sticky. Liquids in the puree consistency should be extremely thick. As per the IDDSI liquids that are extremely thick must sit in a mound or pile above the fork. A small amount may flow through and form a tail below the fork. The liquid or food does not dollop, flow or drip continuously through the fork prongs. Individuals on a puree diet may have their food puree and the liquids may be extremely thick, moderately thick, mildly thick, slightly thick or thin depending on personal needs. A speech language pathologist can test to determine the appropriate texture for foods and liquid by doing a swallowing evaluation.
The degree of severity among individuals with dysphagia can vary from person to person. Individuals should be assessed and prescribed the level of food texture and drink thickness. Physical and cognitive abilities should be taken into consideration with the assessment. The assessment should be comprehensive and may need to be individualized.

This cookbook focuses on puree diets and guidelines for safe swallowing. Remember that dysphagia patients have individual requirements, so these guidelines may not apply to every patient. Consultation with a qualified Speech Language Pathologist or Occupational Therapeutics is recommended to ensure the correct diet consistency is served. A registered dietitian nutritionist can assist in determining the amount of food and liquids to be served. This is important ensure adequate nutrition and fluids are provided. The registered dietitian nutritionist can assess the nutritional needs and develop personalized meal plans.

Warning Signs of Dysphasia:

Report changes immediately to your medical provider.

→Poor dentition, poor gum heath, sores in the mouth or poor mouth care

→Prolonged oral preparatory phase (taking a long time to begin to swallow)

→Needing to swallow 3-4 times for each bite of food

→Coughing

→Frequent throat clearing

→Weak cough (before, during or after a swallow)

→Difficulty controlling liquids in the mouth

→Difficulty controlling mouth secretions

→Wet/gurgled voice

→Pocketing food in the mouth

→Spitting food out

→Extremely slow eater (more than 45 minutes per meal) which is not due to self feeding difficulty

→Giving up or tiring out before the meal is eaten due to extreme fatigue or shortness of breath

→Rocking the tongue back and forth (front to back) also known tongue thrust

→Refusing to eat

→Unexplained loss of appetite

→Repeated upper respiratory infections

→Persistent low grade fever

→Unintentional weight loss or malnutrition

→Recurring or persistent pneumonia

→Fullness of or tightness in throat or chest

→Sensation of food sticking in the throat or sternal area

The Dysphagia Care Team:

Anyone displaying any of the noted signs should be referred to the dysphasia care team: the physician, speech language pathologist, nurse and dietitian for an evaluation. The speech pathologist will assess for problems with dentition, tongue movement, transit of food from the mouth through the esophagus, pocketing of food in the mouth, pooling of liquids and suspected aspiration.

The Speech pathologist may ask the consumer or caregiver the following questions to further assess the dysphasia:

Have you had any recent change in eating habits?

Have you had any recent weight loss?

Do you tend to avoid liquids?

Are liquids hard for you to swallow?

Are you having any difficulty swallowing?

Do you feel like food is stuck in your throat or chest?

Do you tend to clear your throat frequently?

Do you feel a need to swallow 3 or 4 times per bite of food?

Do you cough before during or after swallowing?

Do you have a wet, gurgled or hoarse sounding voice?

The Speech Language Pathologist may also do a physical examine to assess for dysphasia. This may include an assessment of facial weakness, mouth control of food and fluids, impaired motor coordination, strength of the swallowing muscles and function of the nerves in the oral cavity and pharynx. This will determine if further assessment is need.

There are different treatments for various types of dysphasia. First, doctors and **speech-language pathologists** who test for and treat swallowing disorders use a variety of tests that allow them to look at the parts of the swallowing mechanism. One test, called a fiber optic laryngoscopy, allows the doctor to look down the throat with a lighted tube. Other tests, including video fluoroscopy, which takes videotapes of a patient swallowing, and ultrasound, which produces images of internal body organs, can painlessly take pictures of various stages of swallowing.

If the Speech Language pathologist determines it is necessary, further tests will be requested. The most common diagnostic test for dysphasia is the video fluoroscopic swallowing study or modified barium swallow that is needed if conditions exist including but not limited to: abnormal cough, cough after swallow and or voice change after swallow. The video fluoroscopic swallowing study is a moving x-ray of the swallowing process which may be done to determine the type of dysphasia problem that exists and how best to treat it. If the problem originates beyond the pharynx, the video fluoroscopic swallowing study can identify the problem and assist the dysphasia care team in determining the most appropriate interventions. During the video, fluoroscopic swallowing study, the client is videotaped via x-ray machine while consuming small amounts of liquid barium, then pudding and lastly crackers or other foods that require chewing. The Speech Language Pathologist then examines images of the bolus as it moves from the oral cavity and pharynx, structural abnormalities, and or silent aspiration.

Oral dysphasia may be diagnosed if a patient has difficulty initiating a swallow due to difficulty chewing, difficulty manipulating food in the mouth or propelling food to the back of the throat.

Pharyngeal dysphasia may be diagnosed if the bolus penetrates the larynx causing aspiration due to delayed swallow reflux, incomplete closure of the larynx or residence remaining the pharynx after swallow

In esophageal dysphasia food is unable to move easily through the esophagus due esophageal dysmotility, structural blockage, stenosis, or strictures due to GERD. (gastro esophageal reflux)

Treatment:

Once the specific type of dysphasia diagnosed, treatment goals should include:

- Prevention of choking and aspiration
- Maintain good nutritional status and normal weight
- Facilitate or simplify independent eating and swallowing
- Enhance enjoyment of eating
- Enhance quality of life

Once the cause of the dysphasia is found, surgery or medication may help. If treating the cause of the dysphasia does not help, the doctor may have the patient see a speech-language pathologist who is trained in testing and treating swallowing disorders. The speech-language pathologist will test the person's ability to eat and drink and may teach the person new ways to swallow.

Treatment may involve muscle exercises to strengthen weak facial muscles or to improve coordination. For others, treatment may involve learning to eat in a special way. For example, some people may have to eat with their head turned to one side or looking straight ahead. Preparing food in a certain way or avoiding certain foods may help other people. For instance, those who cannot swallow liquids may need to add special thickeners to their drinks. Other people may have to avoid hot or cold foods or drinks.

For some, however, consuming foods and liquids by mouth may no longer be possible. These individuals must use other methods to nourish their bodies. Usually this involves a feeding system, such as a feeding tube, that by passes the part of the swallowing mechanism that is not working normally.

SPECIAL CONSIDERATIONS TO CONSIDER DURING MEALTIMES. YOUR SPEECH LANGUAGE PATHOLOGICS CAN ASSIST WITH YOUR BEST PERSONAL TECHNIQUES.

- Close supervision of individuals with dysphagia closely during meal time is recommended.

- Maintain an upright position (as near 90 degrees as possible) whenever eating or drinking.

- Take small bites -- only 1/2 to 1 teaspoon at a time.

- Eat slowly. It may also help to eat only one food at a time.

- Avoid talking while eating.

- When one side of the mouth is weak, place food into the stronger side of the mouth. At the end of the meal, check the inside of the cheek for any food that may have been pocketed.

- Try turning the head down, tucking the chin to the chest, and bending the body forward when swallowing. This often provides greater swallowing ease and helps prevent food from entering the airway.

- Do not mix solid foods and liquids in the same mouthful and do not "wash foods down" with liquids, unless you have been instructed to do so by the therapist.

- Eat in a relaxed atmosphere, with no distractions.

- Following each meal, sit in an upright position (90-degree angle) for 30 to 45 minutes. regular food. The diets vary in texture and consistency, and are chosen depending on which would be most effective for a specific patient.

General Guidelines for Puree diet: All foods are prepared to a smooth consistency by grinding and then pureeing. Appearance is smooth and cohesive like pudding. The texture of the foods should not be thinner than the prescribed liquid consistency.

1. Watch fluids carefully on individuals who require liquids thickened to nectar, honey or pudding consistency. For some liquids are harder to swallow than solids. Fluids should be allowed at the thickness only. If thin liquids are restricted, avoid milkshakes, frozen yogurt, eggnog, ice cream, sherbet, gelatin or any that are liquid at room temperature unless thickened to correct texture with a thickening agent.
2. Breads and cooked cereals are allowed puree diet plan. The breads and cereals must be processed to a smooth cohesive consistency. (like mashed potatoes.) Milk works well to puree breads and cereals. Breads should be smooth and of one consistency (usually cooked cereals such as cream of wheat or rice or farina) Avoid dry, course, cereals, dry whole grain, cereal with nuts, seeds and coconut. Cereals should have little texture, such as cream of wheat or rice or fine oatmeal. Cream of Wheat or Cream of Rice can be substituted for puree bread.
3. Custards, smooth yogurts, milkshakes, yogurt, milk shakes, eggnogs, ice cream and sherbet are allowed if consistency allowed. Desserts such as pies, cookies, and cakes can be processed to a smooth cohesive consistency. Milk may be added to desserts to process and make a slurry. Avoid bread or rice pudding or any coarse or textured desserts. Avoid desserts with dried fruits, nuts, seeds, coconut or hard to process textures.
4. Fruits and vegetables should be pureed to the proper consistency, with no pulp, tough fibers, seeds, skins or chunks
5. Meats, eggs, cheese and cottage cheese should be pureed. Avoid peanut butter unless part of a complete pureed recipe that is easy to swallow.
6. Menu items should be served individually and not mixed together.
7. All potatoes and other starches should be puree. Mashed potatoes can be served with gravy, sauce, butter or margarine to moisten
8. Soups must be pureed to smooth out any chunks or lumps. To puree soups, strain any chunks or lumps and process until smooth, then add back to broth or liquid.

9. Foods should be served separately and not mixed together in one bowl. Refer to menu or recipes for food items.
10. Avoid other difficult to chew items (nuts, large edible seeds, popcorn, potato or corn chips)
11. Avoid:
    - Dry coarse cakes, cookies, skin, nuts, seed, coconut, pineapple, dried fruit, dry and hard or sticky rice or breading, frozen fruit, rice or bread pudding frozen fruit juice bars, fresh or frozen fruits.
    - Dry tough meat, any other whole pieces of meat, cheese slices or cubes, peanut butter sandwiches, or pizza
    - Potato chips, skin, fried or French fried potatoes Avoid sticky rice. Some individuals have difficulty with rice. Cream of rice may be substituted.
    - Soups with large chunks or meats and vegetables, rice corn or peas, Soup fillings should be smooth and cohesive consistency with consistency of liquid broth as ordered
    - Any sticky foods, chewy candies such as peanut butter, caramels, licorice

Food Group	Allowed	Avoid
Fluids	Ordered consistency	Anything outside of ordered consistency Foods that are liquid are room temperature (unless thin liquids are allowed)
Breads, Cereals, Grains	Pureed bread items, starches etc. Fine textured cereals such as cream of rice or cream of wheat Breads may be pureed into other foods Breads may be puree and seasoned with cinnamon and sugar	Anything that is not of a pureed or slurred consistency Chunky Oatmeal other than very smooth or pureed texture. Blend milk well into hot cereal if thin liquids are not allowed. Starches with nuts, seeds, tough skins and tough potato skins. Sticky puree rice – use cream of rice.
Vegetables	Pureed vegetables to a smooth cohesive consistency. Moist Mashed potatoes with gravy, sauce, or butter Tomato or vegetable juice at proper consistency	Anything other than foods listed in "allowed" category. Vegetables with tough skin or strings. Avoid the seeds of vegetables, stringy fibrous hard to process vegetables such as green onions, leeks, chives, artichokes, corn and raw celery. Vegetables with large seeds (whole winter squash, pumpkin)
Fruits	Pureed to a smooth cohesive consistency with no seeds, pulp, tough skins or chunks. Fruit juice at proper consistency	Anything other than foods listed in "allowed" category. Fruit skin, seeds and dried fruits with tough skins. Watermelon with seeds. Avoid grapes with tough skin and pineapple.
Meat, Fish Poultry or another Protein Foods	Pureed to smooth cohesive consistency with no bone, chunks or lumps.	Anything other than foods listed in "allowed" category. Bacon, tough skin, casing, nuts, grizzle Meat, Fish or Poultry with bones

Meat Substitutes and Casseroles	Pureed according to recipes provided with no chunks or lumps Puree Cottage cheese, cheese, eggs, soups and casseroles must all be pureed	Anything other than foods listed in "allowed" category
Dairy and Milk Products	Smooth pudding, custards or yogurt. Milk allowed by prescribed diet.	Any with nuts, seeds, chunks or other crunchy substances.
Desserts, Snacks, Misc.	Pureed desserts with a smooth cohesive consistency. Smooth Ices, gelatins, frozen juice bars, ice cream, sherbets and milk shakes may only be used if thin liquids are allowed Sugar, salt, sweetened and ground pepper as allowed on therapeutic diets Smooth condiments such as mustard, mayonnaise, ketchup, barbeque sauce, honey, jelly Smooth melt in your mouth candy such as chocolate if thin liquids are allowed and individuals can tolerate	Anything other than foods listed in "allowed" category. Any desserts with course or chunky additives. Hard candy, chewy candy, popcorn, marshmallows, chips, pretzels, raisons
Fats and Oils	Butter, margarine, gravy, cream sauce, mayonnaise, salad dressing cream cheese with puree fruits or puree vegetables added, sour cream, sour cream dips with pureed fruits or vegetables, whipped toppings	All fats with coarse or chunky additives.

Sample Puree

Breakfast	Lunch	Dinner
Orange Juice * Cream of Rice Scrambled Eggs Puree Toast Margarine Milk Coffee * Condiments	Puree Spaghetti with Puree Meatballs Puree Lettuce Salad with Puree Dressing Puree Garlic Bread Puree Peaches Milk * Condiments	Puree Baked Chicken Breast with gravy Puree Sweet Potatoes Puree Broccoli Puree Watermelon Puree Bread Margarine Milk * Condiments

*Note liquids should be thickened to correct consistency.

Thickened Liquids

Individual with dysphasia should be assessed by a speech language pathologist and physician to determine the need for an alteration in the thickness of liquids provided. Thin liquids tend to be more difficult to swallow and can be aspirated easily. Thickening liquids helps slow the transit time through the mouth and pharynx and allows nerve and muscle stimulation. Thickening prevents liquids from falling free and is more easily controlled. **Thickened liquids as recommended by the speech and language pathologist and ordered by the physician will minimize the risk of choking aspiration**.

General Guidelines for Thickened Liquids:
The following consistencies may be ordered based on individual needs:

- **Thin** – water, coffee, tea, soda, ices, juices, milk, anything will liquefy in the mouth within a few seconds
- **Nectar like-** thickened to nectar consistency such as apricot or peach nectar; Liquids have a consistency that coats and drips off a spoon, similar to unset gelatin
- **Honey like-**thickened to honey consistency; The liquid flows off a spoon in a ribbon, just like honey
- **Spoon thick-** thickened to pudding consistency; The liquid remains on the spoon in a soft mass

Be sure to thicken all liquids to the proper consistency including soups, water and all other beverages

Thin	Nectar Like	Honey Like	Spoon thick
Broth, bouillon Carbonated Beverages Coffee Gelatin Ice chips Ice Cream Ices Juices Malts Milk Milkshakes Nutritional supplements Shakes Soda Soups, thin Tea Tomato juice Yogurt, frozen	Apricot nectar Commercial thickeners may be used to achieve nectar like consistency Commercially prepared nectar like thick product Peach nectar Pear nectar Vegetable juice	Commercial product need to achieve desired consistency Commercially prepared honey like thick products	Commercial product needed to achieve desired consistency

Thickened Liquids with IDDSI

IDDSI has developed a method to measure the viscosity of liquids. With this method, liquids are classified based on their rate of flow under the action of gravity down a narrow tube with an opening at the end of the tube. IDDSI has specified the common 10-ml syringe due to its increased availability and affordability globally. Liquids are measured at levels 0-4.

Flow Test Instructions:

Equipment needed: stop watch and 10 ml syringe

1. Remove plunger from syringe and discard
2. Cover the nozzle of the syringe with your finger
3. Fill the syringe with the liquid to the 10 ml line it is recommended you use another 10 ml. syringe to do this)
4. Remove your finger from the nozzle at the same time starting the stop watch.
5. At 10 seconds replace your finger over the nozzle stopping the liquid flowing.

Slightly Thick (Level 1) = 1 ml
Mildly Thick (Level 2) = 4 ml
Moderately Thick (Level 3) = 8 ml or Drips slowly in dollops/strands through prongs of fork
Extremely Thick (Level 4) – do not flow through a 10 ml syringe and are best consumed with a spoon. Fork test and/ or Spoon Tilt Test are recommended methods for determining consistency. For the Fork test the food sits in a mound or pile above the fork. A small amount may flow through and form a tail below the fork. Does not dollop, flow, or drip continuously through the fork prongs.

IDDSI NUMBER	IDSSI LABEL	IDDSI COLOR
7	Regular	Black
6	Soft & Bite -Sized	Blue
5	Minced & Moist	Orange
4	Puree/Extremely Thick	Green
3	Liquidised/ Moderately Thick	Yellow
2	Mildly Thick	Pink
1	Slightly Thick	Grey
0	Thin	White

The International Dysphagia Diet Standardisation Initiative 2016 @ http://iddsi.org/framework/.

LEVELS of Liquids:

THIN	
Description/Characteristics	- Flows like water - Fast flow - Can drink through any type of teat/nipple, cup or straw as appropriate for age and skills
Physiological rationale for this level of thickness	- Functional ability to safely manage liquids of all types
Testing Method	
IDDSI Flow Test*	Test liquid flows through a 10 mL slip tip syringe completely within 10 seconds, leaving no residue (see IDDSI Flow Test instructions*)

SLIGHTLY THICK	
Description/Characteristics	Thicker than water Requires a little more effort to drink than thin liquids Flows through a straw, syringe, teat/nipple Similar to the thickness of commercially available " Anti-regurgitation" (AR) infant formula
Physiological rationale for this level of thickness	Predominately used in the paediatric population as a thickened drink that reduces speed of flow yet is still able to flow through an infant teat/nipple. Consideration to flow through a teat/nipple should be determined on a case-by-case basis.

Testing Method	
IDDSI Flow Test*	Test liquid flows through a 10 mL slip tip syringe leaving 1-4 mL in the syringe after 10 seconds (see IDDSI Flow Test instructions*)

MILDLY THICK	
Description/Characteristics	- Flows off a spoon
- Sippable, pours quickly from a spoon, but slower than thin drinks
- Effort is required to drink this thickness through standard bore straw (standard bore straw = 0.209 inch or 5.3 diameter)
Physiological rationale for this level of thickness	- If thin drinks flow too fast to be controlled safely, these Mildly Thick Liquids will flow at a slightly slower rate
- May be suitable if tongue control is slightly reduced
Testing Method	
IDDSI Flow Test*	- Test liquid flows through a 10 mL slip tip syringe leaving 4-8 mL in the syringe after 10 seconds (see IDDSI Flow Test instructions*)

LIQUIDISED MODERATELY THICK	
Description/Characteristics	- Can be drunk from a cup - Some effort is required to suck through a standard bore or wide bore straw (side bore straw = 0.275 inch or 6.9 mm) - Cannot be piped, layered or moulded on a plate - Cannot be eaten with a fork because it drips slowly in dollops through the prongs - Can be eaten with a spoon - No oral processing or chewing required- can be swallowed directly - Smooth texture with no "bits" (lumps, fibers, bits of shell or skin, husk, particles of gristle or bone)
Physiological rationale for this level of thickness	- If tongue control is insufficient to manage Mildly Thick drinks (Level 2), this liquidized /Moderatley thick level may be suitable - Allows more time for oral control - Needs some tongue propulsion effort - Pain on swallowing

Testing Method	
IDDSI Flow Test*	• Test liquid flows through a 10 mL slip tip syringe leaving > 8 mL in the syringe after 10 seconds (see IDDSI Flow Test instructions*)
Fork Drip Test	• Drips slowly in dollops through the prongs of a fork • Tine/Prongs of a fork do not leave a clear pattern on the surface • Spreads out if spilled onto a flat surface
Spoon Tilt Test	• Easily pours from spoon when tilted; does not stick to spoon
Chopstick Test	• Chopsticks are not suitable for this texture
Finger Test	• It is not possible to hold a sample of this food texture using fingers, however, this texture slides smoothly and easily between the thumb and fingers, leaving a coating
Food Specific or Other examples (NB. This list is not exhaustive)	The Following items may fit into IDDSI Level 3: • Infant "first foods" (runny rice cereal or runny pureed fruit) • Sauces and gravies • Fruit syrup

PUREED/ EXTREMELY THICK	
Description/ Characteristics	- Usually eaten with a spoon (a fork is possible)
- Cannot be drunk from a cup
- Cannot be sucked through a straw
- Does not require chewing
- Can be piped, layered or molded
- Shows some very slow movement under gravity but cannot be poured
- Falls off spoon in a single spoonful when tilted and continues to hold shape on a plate
- No lumps
- Not sticky
- Liquid must me separate from solid
Physiological rationale for this level of thickness	- If tongue control is significantly reduced, this category may be easiest to manage
- Requires less propulsion effort than Minced & Moist (Level 5), Soft & Bite Sized (Level 6) and Regular (Level 7) but more than Liquidized/ Moderately thick (Level 3)
- No biting or chewing is required
- Increased residue is a risk if too sticky
- Any food that requires chewing, controlled manipulation or bolus formation are not suitable
- Pain on chewing or swallowing
- Missing teeth, poorly fitting dentures

Testing Method	
IDDSI Flow Test*	• n/a flow test not applicable, please revert to Fork Drip Test and Spoon Tilt Test
Fork Pressure Test	• The tines/prongs of a fork can make a clear pattern on the surface, and/or the food retains the indentation from the fork • No Lumps
Fork Drip Test	• Sample sits on a mound/pile above the fork; a small amount may flow through and form a tail below the fork tines/prongs, but it does not flow or drip continuously through the prongs of a fork
Spoon Tilt Test	• Cohesive enough to hold its shape on the spoon • A full spoonful must plop off the spoon if the spoon is titled or turned sideways: a very gentle flick may be necessary to dislodge the sample from the spoon, but the sample should slide off easily with very little food left on the spoon; i.e. the sample should not be firm and sticky • May spread out slightly or slump very slowly on a flat plate.
Chopstick test	• Chopsticks are not suitable for this texture
Finger test	• It is just possible to hold a sample of this texture using fingers. • The texture slides smoothly and easily between the fingers and leaves a noticeable residue
Indicators that a sample is too thick	• Does not fall of the spoon when tilted • Sticks to spoon

PREPARATION SUGGESTIONS FOR PUREE DIETS

FOOD ITEM	PUREED TEXTURE GOAL	"HOW TO" TIPS FOR PUREED DIET
Sandwiches	Moist, mashed potatoes.	*Examples:* 1. Puree sandwich filling, and place between pieces of gelled bread. (See Bread below for gelling directions.) 2. Puree bread separately than meat. Serve bread and meat separately. Cream of Wheat can be substituted for the bread on the menu. ½ c. = 1 slice bread. Use whole grain cream of wheat for extra fiber.
Peanut butter sandwiches	None.	**DO NOT PROVIDE**.
Meats, poultry	Puree Like soft, mashed potatoes Free of lumps.	If meat is very dry or stringy, add 1 tsp. vegetable oil, olive oil, liquid margarine, or Broth per 3 oz. serving. Low fat or calorie controlled diets should use broth. You may also need to add 1-2 Tbsp. stabilizer (bread crumbs, xanthan gum or potato flakes) to reach a smooth consistency. Meats tend to require longer processing to achieve mashed potato texture. Process the meat to a ground consistency first and then add the extra oil or broth first slowly until the correct consistency is achieved. Add oil, broth and thickener in small amounts (1 t.) per serving until desired consistency is achieved. *Example:* To each 3-oz. portion of roast beef add 1 tsp. vegetable oil and 1 Tbsp. of the following to thicken: (ONLY ADD THICKENERS IF NEEDED) - Instant food thickener - Instant mashed potato flakes - Dried bread crumbs - Instant cream of wheat or rice Processed meats (bologna, hot dogs, salami) may also need 1-2 tsp. water added. Ham can be very dry, and may need 2-4 Tbsp. water per 3 oz. serving.
Fish	Same as meats & poultry	Because fish is usually very dry, may add 1-2 tsp. vegetable oil, mayonnaise, tartar sauce, or lemon juice for moisture.
Cheese	Smooth, Finely grated; like grated parmesan.	Sprinkle grated parmesan on pureed spaghetti sauce over pureed noodles. Finely shredded cheddar cheese mixed in a pureed tuna casserole. Use cheese sauce or "squeeze cheese" instead of hard cheese for flavor on sandwiches or on gelled crackers for a snack. Use cheese that melt easily and heat until melted. Puree cottage cheese (not the dry curd type) to smooth texture.

Bread	Moist, mashed potatoes.	Bread products do not always puree well. *Alternatives:* 1. Substitute 1/2 c. potatoes or noodles (soft, cooked, mashed) for each slice of bread. 2. Gelled bread, crackers, muffins, other bread products: Make mixture of 1 cup juice, broth, water, syrup (any combination), and 1 1/2 tsp. unflavored gelatin power. Pour 2-4 Tbsp. gelatin/liquid mixture over each slice of bread or another product. Cover (with lid not touching bread). Chill for at least two hours. Result: "Gelled" bread! Can be eaten with a spoon. 3. Menu calls for 1 sl. toast. Substitute 1/2 c. puree oatmeal or other hot cereal. 4. Menu calls for 1 pc. 2" x2" cornbread. Moisten with milk and process to smooth consistency. May gel cornbread, or substitute 1/2 c. polenta or cornmeal mush. 5. Cream of wheat, oatmeal or cream of rice can be substituted for bread on menu.
Noodles (Pasta)	Soft, moist, mashed potatoes	Puree when hot. Puree separately from accompanying food item. May add 1 tsp. margarine per 1/2 c. portion; will also need 2-3 Tbsp. water or milk due to stickiness of pasta. *Example:* Beef Stroganoff: Puree noodles. Then puree meat sauce separately and spoon over pureed noodles. This promotes the appearance of "normal" food.
Rice	Puree smooth and free of lumps	Does not usually puree well; tiny, hard particles will remain that some can't tolerate. Be sure that rice is very well cooked and mash with a fork. Alternatives: For each 1/2 c. of rice on menu, substitute 1/2 c. of quick cooking rice cereal. Some individuals may not tolerate puree rice and cream of rice should be substituted. Example: Rice/chicken casserole Instead of rice, prepare 1/2 c. of rice cereal. Flavor rice cereal with 1 tsp margarine and 1 to 2 Tbsp. of broth or gravy. Puree chicken separately with 1 tsp. margarine and 1 tsp. bread crumbs. Spread pureed chicken over flavored rice cereal for appearance and flavor similar to non- pureed chicken on rice. Flavor Enhancers: Ground/ powder herb and spices may be added to enhance flavor. (Add a dash of cinnamon, paprika, garlic powder etc.) The zest of lemon, lime or orange can also be added to enhance flavor.
Vegetables	Puree Soft, well cooked. Like soft, mashed potatoes. Free of lumps	"Starchy" and "Watery" vegetables puree differently, and require different preparation. 1. "Starchy" (root, tuber) vegetables: (Examples: Potatoes, squash, carrots, yams). To each 1/2 c. portion add 1 tsp. margarine. If consistency is quite stiff and/or dry, add 1 Tbsp. or more of broth, gravy or sauce for softer texture.

		2. "Watery" (leaf, stem, flower) vegetables: (Examples: Green beans, tomatoes, lettuce, spinach and other greens). To each portion add 1-2 tsp. mashed potato flakes or bread crumbs as a stabilizer (to add thickness or "body"), and 1-2 tsp. water. 3. Lettuce: To make lettuce salad or spread, puree 1 c. raw lettuce and other leafy salad ingredients. Add 1/2-1 Tbsp. stabilizer and either 1 1/2 tsp. mayonnaise or neutral colored salad dressing such as Italian or Ranch dressing. May add green food coloring. Can be served as a vegetable or spread on bread for a sandwich.
Fruits	Puree smooth and cohesive or applesauce-like. Free of lumps	Most canned fruits are watery and require a stabilizer. Others have more body and do not require any additions. Examples: - All canned fruits (except applesauce): To each 1/2 c. portion add 1-2 Tbsp. potato flakes or another stabilizer. - Fresh fruit must be soft, ripe and peeled (unpeeled edible peeling if not tough is ok for more fiber) before processing. Use melon, peaches, plums, nectarines, strawberries in season. Add 1-2 Tbsp. stabilizer, depending on water content of fruit. Stabilizers: light cream cheese, nonfat yogurt, sour cream or thickening agents. No grapes, oranges or grapefruit - Molded salad: Substitute pureed fruit for part of the water when preparing a fruit/gelatin salad.
Bananas	Puree smooth and cohesive, soft. Free of lumps	To stop browning, add 1/2 tsp. lemon juice to each 1/2 c. of mashed banana. Orange juice is not a good substitute.

* Puree each food item separately. Serve food items separately.

Puree Recipe Principles:
The following are guidelines to assist you in preparing meals.
1. Measure out the correct serving.
2. Drain any excess liquids.
3. Add extra ingredients such as nonfat milk powder, margarine, butter, sugar etc. if trying to increase calories.
4. Only add liquid if needed and add only gradually.
5. Add stabilizer as needed. Only add the required amount to achieve the correct consistency. (add too much can affect the flavor and too much of certain thickeners can contribute to constipation)
6. Measure out the product for the portion.
7. Add seasonings, puree sauces, gravies as a topping is best so the flavor is not lost in the mixture.

Preserving Nutrients in Puree Food Preparation
The key to preserving nutrients in puree foods is to prepare the food in a way that prevents the loss of nutrients. The recommended consistency of puree food is pudding or mashed potato consistency. The prepared products should nutrient dense and in the appropriate serving size. Use of standardized recipes is essential to produce quality puree products. Follow the instructions to preserve nutrients.

Kitchen Equipment and Food Processing Tips

1. Start with the correct equipment. A food processor is usually the best for pureeing foods like meat, vegetables and fruits. For single servings, the smallest size food processor (1-2 cup size) will work best. A blender can also be used but needs to be checked for lumps.
2. Read and follow the manufactures directions.
3. Always cut large pieces of food into smaller pieces.
4. Do not overload the processor or blender. As a rule of thumb, remember that after being processed, food should not reach more than 2/3 of the way up to the central hub of the blade assembly.
5. To puree foods, start with the chop function. Use the pulse action two or three pulses or until pieces are small. Only add liquid if needed. Soft fruits and vegetables may not need extra liquid.
6. To clean, unplug the unit. Rinse the bowl, blade and cover immediately after each use so food do not stick on them. Wash blade assembly, bowl, cover and spatula in warm soapy water. Rinse and dry. Wash the blade carefully.
7. Never leave blade in soapy water where it may disappear from sight. If you have a dishwasher, you can wash the work bowl, cover, blade assembly and spatula on the top rack. Insert the work bowl upside down and the cover right side up. Put the blade and spatula in the cutlery basket. Unload the dishwasher carefully to avoid contact with sharp blade. Wipe the motor base with damp sponge or cloth. Dry it immediately. Never submerge motor base or the plug-in water or other liquid.
8. Occasionally food will stick to the sides of the bowl as you process. Stop the machine to clear food away. AFTER THE BLADE, HAS STOPPED MOVING, remove the cover, and use a spatula to scrape the food from the sides of the bowl back into the center. Never put hands into bowl unless the processor is unplugged.

General Food Safety

1. Always wash hands with warm water and soap for 20 seconds before and after handling food.
2. Always refrigerate perishable foods within 2 hours
3. Cook or freeze fresh poultry, fish, ground meats within 2 days. Other beef, veal, lamb or pork within 3 to 5 days.
4. Perishable foods such as meat poultry should be wrapped securely to maintain quality and prevent meat juices from getting onto other food.
5. To maintain quality when freezing meat and poultry in its original package, wrap the package again with foil or plastic wrap that is recommended for the freezer.
6. Discard cans with dents, rust or is swollen.
7. Do not cross contaminate. Keep raw meat, poultry, fish and their juices away from other foods. After cutting raw meats, wash cutting boards, utensils and counter tops with hot soapy water.
8. Thaw meats in the refrigerator, not at room temperature.
9. Use a thermometer to cook foods to the proper temperature.
10. Hot food should be held at 140 degrees F or warmer.
11. Cold foods should be held at 40 degrees F or colder.
12. Discard any food left out at room temperature for more than 2 hours.
13. Use cooked leftovers within 72 hours.
14. Prepared puree foods can be store in the freezer for up to 30 days.
15. Reheat left overs to 165 degrees F.
16. Discard expired food. Check expiration dates on milk products.

Proper Cooking Temperatures

For safety, be sure foods are cooked to the proper temperature

ITEMS	TEMPERATURE	HOW LONG/GENERAL INFO
COOKING		
Eggs- Served immediately	145° F	For 15 seconds
Eggs- Hot-held for service	155°F	For 15 seconds
Fish and meat not otherwise specified below	145°F	For 15 seconds
Beef, lamb, pork, veal- Chops, cutlets, ribs and steaks	145°F	For 15 seconds
Beef, lamb, pork, veal- Roasts	145°F	For 4 minutes
Ground meats including- Beef, pork, injected and mechanically tenderized Meats, other meats or fish	165°F	For 15 seconds
Poultry or stuffed Fish/meat/pasta/poultry	165°F	For 15 seconds
Food cooked in microwave oven	165°F	Hold covered for 2 minutes after removing

INCREASING CALORIES AND PROTEIN IN MEALS:

Sometimes it is difficult for individuals with dysphagia to get adequate amounts of nourishment and an undesirable weight loss might occur. Supplementing the diet with extra calories and protein may assist with preventing weight loss. For some individuals gaining or maintaining weight is a difficult task. Providing nutrient and calorie dense food options can help.

Food Groups	Tips for increasing calories
Beverages	Use 100% fruit juice or nectar at each meal as a beverage. Add nonfat milk powder to beverage all beverages. Give Instant Breakfast, eggnog or milkshakes as a supplement and add extra milk powder and flavored syrup (choc.) Make hot cocoa with half and half, whipped topping Add honey or sugar and cream to tea and coffee Offer supplements such as ensure plus between meals Drink smoothies with extra ice cream or cream added.
Breads/ Starches	Add extra margarine, butter cream cheese, jelly, or jams to toast, bread, muffins etc. when processing. Add extra margarine, butter and/ or syrup to pancakes, waffles, or French toast when processing Add evaporated milk, nonfat milk powder, brown sugar, sugar or honey to cooked cereals Add extra mayonnaise and avocado or guacamole meats, salads, vegetables. Whip potatoes with half and half and add extra milk powder and margarine or butter. Add extra cheese sauce, cream sauces, sour cream, gravy, catsup, parmesan cheese, butter or margarine to potatoes, rice, or pasta
Meats and Meat Sub.	Add cheese or ricotta cheese and margarine to puree scrambled eggs Add extra cheese, sour cream and salsa to puree eggs Add extra cheese to puree sandwiches Offer Double the meat in sandwiches Top Meat with extra gravy, sauces, catsup or cheese sauce Add extra puree tartar sauce to fish Add Breading to meats before cooking
Fruits	Do not drain liquid from canned fruits Drizzle with powdered sugar or syrup (pancake or chocolate)

Vegetables	Add extra margarine, olive oil, canola oil or butter to cooked vegetables
Top cooked vegetables with cheese sauce
Add ranch dressing to shredded raw vegetables
Serve raw puree vegetables with low fat dip
Add extra salad dressing to puree salad –use creamy dressing for more calories
Make cream soups with half and half or heavy cream
Add peanut butter or cream cheese to celery
Desserts	Add whipped topping to desserts
Drizzle with powdered sugar, brown sugar or syrup
Make gelatin with fruit juice instead of water
Milk and Dairy Products	Use low fat milk and yogurt products
Add milk powder, honey or syrup to milk and yogurts
Add whipped topping and nonfat milk powder to puddings
Make milkshakes with extra milk powder and syrup

What Are Healthy Food Choices?

A healthy eating plan is encouraged. A diet rich in nutrients can influence overall health. A well-planned balanced diet with adequate amounts of nutrients, a variety of foods, and the correct level of calories for energy is essential to maintain good overall health.

Food are grouped into food groups based on nutrient contents.
The Food groups include, Fruits, Vegetables, Grains, Protein foods, Milk and Milk products, oil, and discretionary calories. Foods in each food group have similar nutritional content. All food groups are important. Omitting food groups can lead to malnutrition.

Fruits and Vegetables:
A variety of whole fruits and vegetables should be served each day. Serving and eating more fruits and vegetables is important. Getting enough fruits and vegetables may reduce the risk of many diseases.
All forms of fruits and vegetables matter and should be encouraged: fresh, frozen, canned, and 100% juice. A diet rich in vegetables and fruits provide Vitamin C, folate, Vitamin A, Vitamin E and dietary fiber. Fruit and vegetables contributes fiber to the diet. Diets rich in dietary fiber have been shown to have beneficial effects including decreasing the risk of coronary heart disease and certain types of cancer. Most fruits and vegetables naturally do not contain very much fat. A couple of exceptions include avocados and olives. Most of their fat is unsaturated and are not harmful to heart health.

Fruits and vegetables are rich in potassium, which may help to maintain a healthy blood pressure. Fruits and vegetables are also low in sodium naturally. Fruits and vegetables are a good source of Vitamin A. Vitamin A keeps eyes and skin healthy and helps protect against infections. Fruits and Vegetables are also a good source of Vitamin C. Vitamin C helps heal cuts and wound and keeps teeth and gums healthy.

The Dietary Guidelines for Americans recommends eating more fruits and vegetables than any other food group. Focus on encouraging more consumption of fruits and vegetables.

Fruits and vegetables are rich in Phytochemicals. Phytochemicals have many benefits for the body. Examples include: Lycopene to reduce the risk of prostate cancer; Lutein to prevent heart disease and decrease risk of macular eye degeneration; Beta-Caratene for bone and skin health; Anthocyanidins for blood vessel health; Quercatin commonly found in kale, onions and grapes can reduce inflammations from allergies. Monoterpenes of citrus fruits and cherries can help protect the lung. Some researchers estimate there are up to 4,000 phytochemicals identified by Scientists.

Nutrients are better absorbed in whole food form rather than supplements. Fruits and vegetables are loaded with the nutrients needed daily.

Buy fresh fruits and vegetables in season. Although most fresh fruits and vegetables are now available year around, some are less expensive when they are in season. Take advantage of sales and seasons. Frozen and canned are also acceptable.

Fruits make an excellent dessert. Encourage fruit for the dessert on meal plans. Avoid adding margarine or butter to vegetables when watching calories. Vegetables may be steamed and prepared without extra added fat. For fruit juice encourage only 100% fruit juice. Since fruit juice does not contain as much fiber as whole fruit and when consumed in large amounts can contribute to extra calories

Do NOT use fruit drinks as fruit servings. Canned fruits should NOT be packed in syrup because they contain too much added sugar if you are watching calories. Canned fruits should be packed in fruit juice without extra sugar added. Canned fruit that is packed in syrup can be rinsed to avoid excess sugar

Food Guide: Fruits

Food Guides:	Consume a variety of fruits
Major Nutrient Contributions:	Folate, Vitamin A, Vitamin C, Potassium and Fiber
Serving Sizes ½ c. puree	1/2c. fruit is equivalent to 1/2 c. fresh, frozen or canned fruit
Best Choices	Apples, apricots, bananas, blueberries, cantaloupe, cherries, grapefruit, grapes, guava, kiwi, melons, mango, nectarines, oranges, papaya, peaches, pears, plums, raspberries, strawberries, tangerines, watermelon
Choices to Avoid or use only on occasion	Canned or frozen fruit packed in syrup; juices, punches, ades, and fruit drinks with added sugars, fried plantains

Vegetables

Food Guides:	Choose a variety of vegetables each day, and choose from all subgroups several times a week
Major Nutrient Contributions:	Folate, Vitamin A, Vitamin C, Vitamin K, Vitamin E, magnesium, potassium and fiber
Serving Sizes	1 c. vegetable serving is equivalent to 1 c. cut up raw or ½ c. cooked vegetables; 2 c. raw leafy greens, Portion size for puree is ½ cup.
Best Choices (a variety of each group each week)	Dark green vegetables: Broccoli and leafy greens such as arugula, beet greens, Bok choy, collard greens, kale, mustard greens, romaine lettuce, spinach and turnip greens Orange and deep yellow vegetables: Carrots, carrot juice, pumpkin, sweet potatoes, and winter squash (acorn, butternut) Other vegetables: Artichokes, asparagus, bamboo shoots, beans sprouts, beets, Brussels sprouts, cabbages, cactus, cauliflower, celery, cucumber, eggplant, green beans, ice berg lettuce, mushrooms, okra, onions, peppers, seaweed, snow peas, tomatoes, vegetable juice, zucchini
Choices to Avoid or use only on occasion	Baked Beans, candied sweet potatoes, coleslaw, French fries, potato salad, refried beans, scalloped potatoes, tempura vegetables

Lean Meats and Protein Sources:

Protein Means "Of Prime Importance"

Protein means "of prime importance". Without protein, your bones, hair, and skin would have no structure. Lacking adequate protein may lead to impaired bodily functions. Your red blood cells will not be able to clot. Your body would not be able to defend against infections. Protein is vital for so many of your basic functions.

Examples of Functions of Protein in your body:

Growth and maintenance
Protein is required daily for growth and maintenance. Each integral part of your body is either, growing, repairing or maintaining. For this your skin, muscles, organs, and bones need much more protein. Children and women who are pregnant have an increased need for protein during growth.

Enzymes
Proteins are necessary to produce enzymes. Enzymes can aid in chemical reactions within our body. Digestive enzymes are just one type of enzyme found in your body. Digestive enzymes assist in breaking down food during digestion.

Hormones
Many hormones are made up of proteins. Hormones assist your body in regulating body processes. Insulin is an example of a hormone produced in your body

Fluid Balance
Proteins are necessary for fluid balance. Inadequate protein can result in the body's lack of ability to move fluids in and out of cells. When fluids build up in excess amount inside the cell it may cause edema.

Acid-base balance
Proteins are necessary to maintain the body's proper acid-base balance. An example of improper balance of acid-balance would be the body's ability to maintain its blood system in the proper acid-balance base. Without the proper balance of acid-balance in the blood system the body could go into acidosis or alkalosis. Both can lead to coma and death.

Transportation
Proteins often work as transporters within the body. Lipids, vitamins, minerals and oxygen all use transporters to circulate within the body.

Antibodies
Proteins are necessary to build antibodies. Antibodies work to protect our bodies against foreign invaders. Without adequate protein, our bodies' resistance to protect against infection is decreased.

Energy and Glucose
Proteins do provide our body with some fuel. Excess protein can be converted to glucose to be used for energy.

Recommended Intakes of Protein.

The protein RDA for adults is .8 grams per kilogram of a HEALTHY body weight person. Individual protein needs may be difficult to establish and may require the assistance of a Registered Dietitian.

The right amount of protein for many people may be altered due to their current nutritional status. Factors that might affect protein requirements include:
Age
Weight
Body Composition
Skin Condition
Infection
Cancer
And so much more....

Meat, Poultry, Fish, Legumes, Eggs and Nuts

Food Guides:	Make lean or low fat choices. Prepare with little or no added fat. Choose seafood 8 oz. a week such as salmon, tuna or herring which are high in Omega 3 fatty acids
Best Choices	Poultry without the skin (skin can be removed after cooking), fish, shellfish, legumes, eggs, lean meat with fat trimmed, low fat tofu; tempeh,
Choices to Avoid or use on occasion	Bacon, baked beans, fried meat, fish, poultry, eggs or tofu; refried beans, ground beef, hot dogs, luncheon meats; marbled steaks; poultry with skin; sausages, spare ribs
Major Nutrient Contribution	Protein, essential fatty acids, niacin, thiamin, vitamin B 12, iron, magnesium, potassium and zinc

Grains:

Grains

Food Guides:	Make at least half of the grains selections whole grains.
Best Choices	Whole grains such as amaranth, barley, brown rice, buckwheat, bulgur, millet, oats, quinoa, rye and wheat; Low fat breads, cereals, crackers and pastas Enriched bagels, breads, cereals, pastas (couscous, macaroni, spaghetti) pretzels, rice, rolls, tortillas
Choices to Avoid or use on occasion	Biscuits, cakes, cookies, cornbread, crackers, croissants, doughnuts, French toast, fried rice, granola, muffins, pancakes, pastries, pies, pre-sweetened cereals, taco shells, waffles
Major Nutrient Contributions	Folate, niacin, riboflavin, thiamin, iron, magnesium, selenium and fiber

Milk and Dairy Products:

Food Guides:	Make fat free or low fat choices. Choose lactose free products or other calcium rich foods if you don't consume milk
Best Choices	Fat free and fat free milk products such as buttermilk, cheese, cottage cheese, yogurt; fat free fortified soy milk; (look for yogurt and pudding that are less than 100 kcal per serving)
Choices to Avoid or use on occasion	Cheese; 1 % low fat milk, 2 % reduced fat milk and whole milk; low fat, reduced fat and whole milk products such as cheese, cottage cheese, and yogurt; milk products with added sugars such as chocolate milk, custard, ice cream, ice milk, milk shakes, pudding, sherbet, fortified soy milk
Major Nutrient Contributions	Protein, riboflavin, Vitamin B 12, calcium, potassium, and when fortified Vitamin A and D

TIPS to SAVE Calories:
Serve Nonfat or Low Milk 3 X daily or 3 cups a day
Serve Yogurt: use fat free sugar free variety approximately 100 or less calories per servings
Cottage Cheese: Serve low-fat cottage cheese
Pudding: May serve fat free and/or sugar free only-look for 100 kcal per serving
Ice Cream: May serve low-fat or fat free sugar free only- look for 100 kcal per serving
Cheese: May choose low-fat varieties – approximately 80 calories per 1 oz. serving.
Sour cream: May low-fat (light on label)
Cream Cheese: May use low-fat (light on label)
Limit the amounts of fats and oils.

Fats and Oils

Best Choices	Use in small amounts. Liquid oils such as olive, canola, corn, flaxseed, nut, peanut and safflower, sesame, soybean, sunflower oils, mayonnaise, oil based salad dressings, soft trans fat free margarine, unsaturated oils that occur naturally in foods like fatty fish, avocados, fatty fish, nuts, olives
Limited of amounts of solid fats	Butter, animal fats, stick margarine, shortening

TIPS: Fats and oils are not a food group but should be included because they contribute Vitamin E and essential oils to the diet. Liquid oils should be used instead of solid fats when possible.
Salad Dressing; Fat Free and reduced fat salad dressings can be served
Mayonnaise: fat free or low fat or light mayonnaise can be served
Margarine and butter should be limited to 1 t. per serving. (about the size of a postage stamp)
Avoid fats with Trans fat in the ingredients.

How much food to serve?

The amount of food to serve can very from person to person depending many factors. Calorie needs depend on:

Body size
Age
Height
Weight
Activity Level
Gender

Other conditions such as neurological disorders, muscle tone, cancer, pressure injuries, (bed sores), burns, fractures, or recent surgeries can also affect caloric needs.

A registered dietitian nutritionist can assist in determining the caloric needs.

Sample Adult Meal Plans Number of Servings:

	Meal	Small 1400-1800 kcal.	Regular 1800-2200 kcal.	Large 2200-2600 kcal.	X-Large 2600-3000 kcal.
	Breakfast				
Grains		1	2	3	3
Vegetables		0	0	0	0
Fruits		1	1	1	2
Dairy		1	1	1	1
Protein		1	1	2	2
	Lunch				
Grains		2	2	4	4
Vegetables		1-3	2-3	2-3	2-3
Fruits		1	1	1	2
Dairy		0	0	0	0
Protein		2	2	4	4
	Dinner				
Grains		1	2	3	3
Vegetables		1-2	1-2	1-2	1-2
Fruits		1	1	1	2
Dairy		1	1	1	1
Protein		3	3	3	4
	Snacks				
Dairy		1	1	1	1
Grains		1	1	1	2

BASIC MEAL PLANS SMALL PORTION DIET 1400 – 1800 KCAL

FOOD GROUP	Servings	Serving Size	Kcal Range
Meat (lean), Poultry, Fish, Dry Beans, Eggs, & Nuts	5 – 6 ounces	1 oz. cooked meat or poultry; 1 egg; 1/4 cup cooked dry beans or tofu	275 -330 kcal
Grains Bread, Cereal, Rice, & Pasta (at least 1/2 of all grains should be whole grains)	3 – 5 servings	1 slice bread; 3/4-1 cup ready-to-eat cereal; 1/2 cup cooked cereal, rice or pasta	240 – 400 kcal
Vegetables (including dark green or deep yellow as a source of vitamin A at least every other day)	5 –6 servings	1 cup raw leafy vegetables; 1/2 cup of other vegetables (raw or cooked); 1/2- 3/4 cup vegetable juice or ½ cup puree	125 –150 kcal
Fruits (at least 1 should be high in vitamin C)	3 servings	1 medium apple, banana, orange, pear; 1/2 cup puree, cooked or canned fruit; 1/2- 3/4 cup fruit juice	180 kcal
Milk, Yogurt, & Cheese (low-fat)	2 ½- 3 servings	1 cup milk or yogurt; 1 1/2 oz. natural cheese; 2 oz. processed cheese	225 – 270 kcal
Fats & Oils	4-6 serving	1 tsp margarine, oil, butter, mayonnaise; 1 TB. regular salad dressing	180-270 kcal
Discretionary Calories*			175-200 kcal
Total Calories			1400 – 1800 kcal

*Calories remaining after the recommended servings from each food group have been met through the consumption of nutrient dense foods. Calories may come from foods such as jelly, sugar, syrup or dessert

BASIC MEAL PLANS LARGE DIET 2200 – 2600 KCAL

FOOD GROUP	Servings	Serving Size	Kcal Range
Meat (lean), Poultry, Fish, Dry Beans, Eggs, & Nuts	9 – 10 ounces	1 oz. cooked meat or poultry; 1 egg; 1/4 cup cooked dry beans or tofu;	495 – 550 kcal
Grains Bread, Cereal, Rice, & Pasta (at least 1/2 of all grains should be whole grains)	8– 10 servings	1 slice bread; 3/4-1 cup ready-to-eat cereal; 1/2 cup cooked cereal, rice or pasta	640 – 800 kcal
Vegetables (including dark green or deep yellow as a source of vitamin A at least every other day)	6 servings	1 cup raw leafy vegetables; 1/2 cup of other vegetables (raw or cooked); 1/2- 3/4 cup vegetable juice or ½ cup puree	150 kcal
Fruits (at least 1 should be high in vitamin C)	5-6 servings	1 medium apple, banana, orange, pear; 1/2 cup chopped, cooked or canned fruit; 1/2-3/4 cup fruit juice	300-360 kcal
Milk, Yogurt, & Cheese (low-fat)	3 servings	1 cup milk or yogurt; 1 1/2 oz. natural cheese; 2 oz. processed cheese	270 kcal
Fats & Oils	5-7 servings	1 tsp margarine, oil, butter, mayonnaise; 1 TB. regular salad dressing	225-315 kcal
Discretionary Calorie Allowance*			120 – 155 kcal
Total Calories			2200 – 2600 kcal

*Calories remaining after the recommended servings from each food group have been met through the consumption of nutrient dense foods. Calories may come from foods such as jelly, sugar, syrup or dessert

BASIC MEAL PLAN EXTRA LARGE DIET 2600 – 3000 KCAL

FOOD GROUP	Servings	Serving Size	Kcal Range
Meat (lean), Poultry, Fish, Dry Beans, Eggs, & Nuts	10 – 11 ounces	1 oz. cooked meat or poultry; 1 egg; 1/4 cup cooked dry beans or tofu	550 – 770 kcal
Grains Bread, Cereal, Rice, & Pasta (at least 1/2 of all grains should be whole grains)	10 – 11 servings	1 slice bread; 3/4- 1 cup ready-to-eat cereal; 1/2 cup cooked cereal, rice or pasta	800 -880 kcal
Vegetables (including dark green or deep yellow as a source of vitamin A at least every other day)	6 servings	1 cup raw leafy vegetables; 1/2 cup of other vegetables (raw or cooked); 1/2- 3/4 cup vegetable juice	150 kcal
Fruits (at least 1 should be high in vitamin C)	5-6 servings	1 medium apple, banana, orange, pear; 1/2 cup chopped, cooked or canned fruit; 1/2-3/4 cup fruit juice	300-360 kcal
Milk, Yogurt, & Cheese (low-fat)	3 servings	1 cup milk or yogurt; 1 1/2 oz. natural cheese; 2 oz. processed cheese	270 kcal
Fats & Oils	6 -7 servings	1 tsp margarine, oil, butter, mayonnaise; 1 TB. regular salad dressing	270-315 kcal
Discretionary Calorie Allowance*			260 – 300 kcal
Total Calories			2600 – 3000 kcal

*Calories remaining after the recommended servings from each food group have been met through the consumption of nutrient dense foods. Calories may come from foods such as jelly, sugar, syrup or dessert.

Common Portions Sizes for Puree Foods

Meat (lean), Poultry, Fish, Dry Beans, Eggs, & Nuts

1 oz. = ¼ cup

2 oz. = 1/3 cup

3 oz. = ½ cup

Grains Bread, Cereal, Rice, & Pasta (at least 1/2 of all grains should be whole grains)

 ½ cup puree

Vegetables (including dark green or deep yellow as a source of vitamin A at least every other day)

½ cup cooked.
1 cup raw to process to about ½ cup with dressing or other sauce.

Fruits (at least 1 should be high in vitamin C)
½ cup
Milk, Yogurt, & Cheese (low-fat)
1 cup milk
2/3 cup yogurt
2 oz. cheese

Fats & Oils
Usually 1 teaspoons but may vary

Sauces
2 tablespoons

Recipes

Beverages:

In this collection of recipes, you will find a variety of smoothies and delicious beverages. The beverages are an excellent way to nourish the body with essential nutrients. For individuals needing thickened liquids the beverages can be further thickened with thickening products to the correct consistency.

Recipe Name: **Banana Berry Fruit Smoothie**
Portion Size: 1 ½ cup
Servings: 1
Ingredients:
1/4 cup nonfat milk (to add extra calories, use whole milk, half and half or cream)
½ banana
½ cup fresh or frozen strawberries
¾ cup nonfat or low fat yogurt (use strawberry, vanilla or plain Greek yogurt)
1 teaspoon honey (optional)
Directions:
In a blender, combine all the ingredients. Blend until smooth

Recipe Name: **Berry Pineapple Fruit Smoothie**
Portion Size: 1 1/2 cup
Servings:1
Ingredients:
1/4 cup nonfat milk (to add extra calories, use whole milk, half and half or cream)
1/4 cup pineapple
1/4 cup fresh or frozen mixed berries
¾ cup nonfat or low fat yogurt (use strawberry, vanilla or plain Greek yogurt)
1 teaspoon honey (optional)
Directions:
In a blender, combine all the ingredients. Blend until smooth

Recipe Name: **Chocolate Banana Smoothie**
Portion Size: 1 cup
Servings: 1
Ingredients:
1/4 cup nonfat milk (to add extra calories, use whole milk, half and half or cream)
1/2 banana
1/2 teaspoon honey (optional)
2 tablespoons chocolate syrup
¾ cup nonfat or low fat yogurt (use vanilla or plain Greek yogurt)
Directions:
In a blender, combine all the ingredients. Blend until smooth

Recipe Name: **Fruited Yogurt Drink**
Portion Size: 1 cup
Servings 1
Ingredients:
1/2 banana
¼ cup peaches or strawberries (fresh, canned or frozen)
2 tablespoons nonfat milk (to add extra calories, use whole milk, half and half or cream)
½ cup nonfat or low fat yogurt (use strawberry, vanilla or plain Greek yogurt)
2 ice cubes
Directions:
In a blender, combine all the ingredients. Blend until smooth

Recipe Name: **High Protein Milk**
Portion Size: 1 cup
Servings: 1
Ingredients:
1 cup nonfat or low fat milk (to add extra calories, use whole milk, half and half or cream)
2 tablespoons Nonfat milk powder
2 tablespoons flavoring (like chocolate or strawberry syrup)
Directions:
In a blender, combine all the ingredients. Blend until smooth.

Recipe Name: **Mango Banana Smoothie**

Portion Size: 1 ½ cup

Servings: 1

Ingredients:

1/4 cup nonfat milk (to add extra calories, use whole milk, half and half or cream)

1/2 banana

1/2 teaspoon honey (optional)

1/2 cup frozen or fresh mango

¼ cup orange mango juice blend

¾ cup nonfat or low fat yogurt (use vanilla or plain Greek yogurt)

Directions:

In a blender, combine all the ingredients. Blend until smooth

Recipe Name: **Raspberry Peach Smoothie**

Portion Size: 1 ½ cup

Servings: 1

Ingredients:

1/4 cup nonfat milk (to add extra calories, use whole milk, half and half or cream)

½ cup fresh, frozen or canned peaches

½ cup fresh or frozen raspberry

¾ cup nonfat or low fat yogurt (use Raspberry, vanilla or plain Greek yogurt)

1 teaspoon honey (optional)

Directions:

In a blender, combine all the ingredients. Blend until smooth

Recipe Name: **Orange Breakfast Sipper**

Portion Size: 1 ½ cup

Servings: 1

Ingredients:

1 cup buttermilk

½ cup frozen orange juice concentrate

1 tablespoon brown sugar or honey

4 ice cubes

Directions:

In a blender, combine all the ingredients. Blend until smooth

Recipe Name: **Orange Frosty**
Portion Size: 1 cup
Servings: 1 1/2 cup
Ingredients:
¼ cup frozen orange juice concentrate
¾ cup milk (to add extra calories, use whole milk, half and half or cream)
¼ cup nonfat milk powder
4 ice cubes
1 teaspoon sugar
¼ teaspoon vanilla
Directions:
In a blender, combine all the ingredients. Blend until smooth

Recipe Name: **Papaya Strawberry Smoothie**
Portion Size: 1 ½ cup
Servings: 1
Ingredients:
1/4 cup nonfat milk (to add extra calories, use whole milk, half and half or cream)
1/4 cup fresh, or frozen papaya pieces
1/4 cup fresh or frozen strawberries
¾ cup nonfat or low fat yogurt (use strawberry, vanilla or plain Greek yogurt)
½ banana
2 ice cubes
Directions:
In a blender, combine all the ingredients. Blend until smooth

Recipe Name: **Peanut Butter Banana Smoothie**
Portion Size: 1 ½ cup
Servings: 1
Ingredients:
1/4 cup nonfat milk (to add extra calories, use whole milk, half and half or cream)
¼ cup Peanut Butter
½ Banana
1 cup nonfat or low fat yogurt (use vanilla or plain Greek yogurt)
1 teaspoon honey (optional)
Directions:
In a blender, combine all the ingredients. Blend until smooth

Recipe Name: **Pina Colada Smoothie**
Portion Size: 1 ½ cup
Servings: 1
Ingredients:
1/4 cup nonfat milk (to add extra calories, use whole milk, half and half or cream)
¼ cup frozen pineapple juice concentrate
½ Banana
1 cup nonfat or low fat yogurt (use vanilla yogurt)
1 teaspoon coconut extract
Directions:
In a blender, combine all the ingredients. Blend until smooth

Recipe Name: **Pineapple Banana Sipper**
Portion Size: 1 ½ cup
Servings: 1
Ingredients:
1/4 cup nonfat milk (to add extra calories, use whole milk, half and half or cream)
¼ cup frozen pineapple juice concentrate
½ Banana
1 cup nonfat or low fat yogurt (use vanilla or plain Greek yogurt)
1 teaspoon honey (optional)
½ teaspoon vanilla extract
Directions:
In a blender, combine all the ingredients. Blend until smooth

Recipe Name: **Pudding Milkshakes**
Portion Size: 1 ½ cup
Servings: 1
Ingredients:
1/4 cup nonfat milk (to add extra calories, use whole milk, half and half or cream)
¼ cup instant pudding mix (any flavor)
1 cup vanilla ice cream
Directions:
In a blender, combine all the ingredients. Blend until smooth

Recipe Name: **Pumpkin Banana Smoothie**
Portion Size: 1 ½ cup
Servings: 1
Ingredients:
1/4 cup nonfat milk (to add extra calories, use whole milk, half and half or cream)
¼ cup Pumpkin puree (may use canned)
½ Banana
1 cup nonfat or low fat yogurt (use vanilla or plain Greek yogurt)
1 tablespoon brown sugar
1 teaspoon vanilla
Directions:
In a blender, combine all the ingredients. Blend until smooth

Recipe Name: **Raspberry Banana Smoothie**
Portion Size: 1 ½ cup
Servings: 1
Ingredients:
1/4 cup nonfat milk (to add extra calories, use whole milk, half and half or cream)
¼ cup Fresh or Frozen raspberries
½ Banana
1 cup firm tofu
2 tablespoons orange juice
1 teaspoon honey
Directions:
In a blender, combine all the ingredients. Blend until smooth

Recipe Name: **High Calorie High Protein Shakes**
Portion Size: 1 ½ cup
Servings: 1
Ingredients:
½ cup half and half
½ cup egg substitute
½ cup ice cream
2 tablespoons sugar
1 teaspoon vanilla
Directions:
In a blender, combine all the ingredients. Blend until smooth

Recipe Name: **Tofu Fruit Smoothie**
Portion Size: 1 ½ cup
Servings: 1
Ingredients:
1/4 cup dessert tofu
¼ cup Fresh or Frozen strawberries
½ cup frozen, fresh or canned peaches.
½ cup nonfat or low fat yogurt (any flavor)
1 teaspoon Orange juice
Directions:
In a blender, combine all the ingredients. Blend until smooth

Breads

Recipe Name: **Banana Bread in a Mug**
Portion Size: 1 mug
Servings:1
Ingredients:
3 tablespoons all purpose flour
1 tablespoon sugar
¼ teaspoon baking powder
pinch salt
¼ teaspoon vanilla
1 ripe mashed ripe bananas
1 tablespoon margarine or butter, softened
1 tablespoon sour cream
2 tablespoons milk (or more for pureeing)
1 egg
Cooking spray
Whipped topping for garnish (optional)
Directions:
In a bowl, mix the banana, eggs, vanilla and sour cream. Slowly stir in the flour, sugar, baking powder, add salt. Mix until combined. Spray microwave safe coffee mug with non-stick cooking spray. Pour into mug. Microwave on high for 2 to 3 minutes. To test for doneness, insert a clean toothpick into the center. If the toothpick comes out clean it is done. Cooking times will vary depending on microwave. Adding 1 teaspoon milk at a time, blend until smooth and consistency of mashed potatoes. Scoop onto serving dish and top with whipped topping.

Recipe Name: **Pumpkin Bread in a Mug**
Portion Size: 1 mug
Servings:1
Ingredients:
¼ cup all purpose flour
2 tablespoons sugar
2 tablespoons pumpkin puree
1/8 teaspoon baking powder
1 tablespoon vegetable oil
pinch salt
pinch of pumpkin spice
¼ teaspoon vanilla
1 tablespoon margarine or butter, softened
2 tablespoons milk (or more for pureeing)
Cooking spray
Whipped topping for garnish (optional)
Directions:
In a bowl, mix the pumpkin, vanilla and oil. Slowly stir in the flour, sugar, baking powder, pumpkin spice and salt. Mix until combined. Spray microwave safe coffee mug with non-stick cooking spray. Pour into mug Microwave on high for 2 to 3 minutes. To test for doneness, insert a clean toothpick into the center. If the toothpick comes out clean it is done. Cooking times will vary depending on microwave. Adding 1 teaspoon milk at a time, blend until smooth and consistency of mashed potatoes. Scoop onto serving dish and top with whipped topping.

Recipe Name: **Pear Bread in a Mug**
Portion Size: 1 mug
Servings: 1
Ingredients:
¼ **cup all purpose flour**
2 tablespoons sugar
3 tablespoons puree canned pears
1/8 teaspoon baking powder
1 tablespoon vegetable oil
pinch salt
¼ teaspoon cinnamon
¼ teaspoon vanilla
1 tablespoon margarine or butter, softened
2 tablespoons milk (or more for pureeing)
Cooking spray
Whipped topping for garnish (optional)
Directions:
In a bowl, mix the puree pears, vanilla and oil. Slowly stir in the flour, sugar, baking powder, cinnamon and salt. Mix until combined. Spray microwave safe coffee mug with non-stick cooking spray. Pour into mug. Microwave on high for 2 to 3 minutes. To test for doneness, insert a clean toothpick into the center. If the toothpick comes out clean it is done. Cooking times will vary depending on microwave. Adding 1 teaspoon milk at a time, blend until smooth and consistency of mashed potatoes. Scoop onto serving dish and top with whipped topping.

Recipe Name: **Apple Bread in a Mug**
Portion Size: 1 mug
Servings: 1
Ingredients:
¼ cup all purpose flour
2 tablespoons sugar
¼ cup applesauce
1/8 teaspoon baking powder
1 tablespoon vegetable oil
pinch salt
¼ teaspoon cinnamon
¼ teaspoon vanilla
1 tablespoon margarine or butter, softened
2 tablespoons milk (or more for pureeing)
Cooking spray
Whipped topping for garnish (optional)
Directions:
In a bowl, mix the puree applesauce, vanilla and oil. Slowly stir in the flour, sugar, baking powder, cinnamon and salt. Mix until combined. Spray microwave safe coffee mug with non-stick cooking spray. Pour into mug. Microwave on high for 2 to 3 minutes. To test for doneness, insert a clean toothpick into the center. If the toothpick comes out clean it is done. Cooking times will vary depending on microwave. Adding 1 teaspoon milk at a time, blend until smooth and consistency of mashed potatoes. Scoop onto serving dish and top with whipped topping.

Desserts

Desserts can be added to meals to add extra calories when needed. Fruit is recommended for dessert but an occasional brownie or cake is a treat! In the dessert section are single quick serving recipes for one prepared in a mug. Desserts should be soft and moist. Desserts should not be sticky. Moisten with milk and stir to a smooth cohesive consistency. Enjoy!

Recipe Name: **Brownie in a Mug**
Portion Size: 1 mug
Servings:1
Ingredients:
4 tablespoons all purpose flour
4 tablespoons sugar
2 tablespoons cocoa powder
2 tablespoon vegetable oil
2 tablespoons water
2 tablespoons milk (or more for pureeing)
Cooking spray
Whipped Topping (optional)
Directions:
In a bowl, mix the flour, sugar, cocoa powder, water and oil. Mix until combined. Spray microwave safe coffee mug with non-stick cooking spray. Pour into mug. Microwave on high for 1 to 3 minutes. To test for doneness, insert a clean toothpick into the center. If the toothpick comes out clean it is done. Cooking times will vary depending on microwave. Adding 1 teaspoon milk at a time, blend until smooth and consistency of mashed potatoes.

Recipe Name: **Chocolate Cake in a Mug**
Portion Size: 1 mug
Servings:1
Ingredients:
¼ cup all purpose flour
2 tablespoons sugar
2 tablespoons cocoa
1/4 teaspoon baking powder
1/8 teaspoon salt
2 tablespoons vegetable oil
¼ cup + 1 tablespoon milk (or more for pureeing)
Cooking spray
Frosting:
¼ cup powdered sugar
1 tablespoon baking cocoa powder,
1 tablespoon milk
¼ teaspoon vanilla
Directions:
In a bowl, mix the ¼ cup + 1 tablespoon milk and oil. Slowly stir in the flour, ¼ cup sugar, baking powder, cocoa and salt. Mix until combined. Spray microwave safe coffee mug with non-stick cooking spray. Pour into mug. Microwave on high for 2 to 3 minutes. To test for doneness, insert a clean toothpick into the center. If the toothpick comes out clean it is done. Cooking times will vary depending on microwave. Adding 1 teaspoon milk at a time, blend until smooth and consistency of mashed potatoes.
For frosting: Combine powdered sugar, baking cocoa, milk and vanilla. Top cake with frosting.

Recipe Name: **Lemon Cake in a Mug**
Portion Size: 1 mug
Servings:1
Ingredients:
6 tablespoons all purpose flour
¼ cup sugar plus 3 tablespoons sugar
1/8 teaspoon baking powder
1 egg
1 tablespoon vegetable oil
2 tablespoons water
1 tablespoon lemon juice plus 1 tablespoon lemon juice
pinch salt
1 tablespoon margarine or butter, softened
2 tablespoons milk (or more for pureeing)
Cooking spray
Directions:
In a bowl, mix the egg, 1 tablespoon, water, lemon juice and oil. Slowly stir in the flour, ¼ cup sugar, baking powder, and salt. Mix until combined. Spray microwave safe coffee mug with non-stick cooking spray. Pour into mug. Microwave on high for 2 1/2 to 3 minutes. To test for doneness, insert a clean toothpick into the center. If the toothpick comes out clean it is done. Cooking times will vary depending on microwave. Adding 1 teaspoon milk at a time, blend until smooth and consistency of mashed potatoes. Mixed 3 tablespoons white sugar and 1 tablespoon lemon juice together in microwave safe bowl. Cook until sauce is bubbling, about 30 seconds. Pour sauce over cake. Scoop onto serving dish and top with lemon sauce.

Recipe Name: **Peanut Butter Cookie in a Mug**
Portion Size: 1 mug
Servings:1
Ingredients:
3 tablespoons all purpose flour
1 tablespoon sugar
1 tablespoon brown sugar
1 egg
1/4 teaspoon baking powder
2 tablespoon butter, softened
1 tablespoon vanilla
6 tablespoons milk (or more for pureeing)
pinch salt
2 tablespoons margarine or butter, softened
Cooking spray
Directions:
Spray microwave safe mug with non-stick cooking spray. Place 1 tablespoon butter butter and peanut butter in a microwave safe mug. Microwave until butter and peanut butter are melted, about 30 seconds. Stir in brown sugar, white sugar, and salt into butter mixture. Add egg and stir. Add flour and stir. Top with remaining 1 tablespoon butter. Microwave on high for 2 1/2 to 3 minutes. To test for doneness, insert a clean toothpick into the center. If the toothpick comes out clean it is done. Cooking times will vary depending on microwave. Adding 1 teaspoon milk at a time, blend until smooth and consistency of mashed potatoes.

Recipe Name: **Vanilla Cake in a Mug**
Portion Size: 1 mug
Servings:1
Ingredients:
6 tablespoons all purpose flour
2 tablespoons sugar
1/4 teaspoon baking powder
2 tablespoon butter, softened
1 tablespoon vanilla
6 tablespoons milk (or more for pureeing)
pinch salt
Cooking spray
Directions:
In a bowl, mix the butter, milk, and oil. Slowly stir in the flour, sugar, baking powder, vanilla and salt. Mix until combined. Spray microwave safe coffee mug with non-stick cooking spray. Pour into mug. Microwave on high for 2 1/2 to 3 minutes. To test for doneness, insert a clean toothpick into the center. If the toothpick comes out clean it is done. Cooking times will vary depending on microwave. Adding 1 teaspoon milk at a time, blend until smooth and consistency of mashed potatoes. Mixed 3 tablespoons white sugar and 1 tablespoon lemon juice together in microwave safe bowl.

Entrees

Meats and Protein Sources:

Meats and Protein sources provide protein to a balanced diet. Meats provide protein which is vital for many basic body functions. Despite's meat's importance puree meat is the most commonly refused puree product. Special attention in the preparation of meat and protein sources should be followed to enhance flavor, acceptance and preserve nutrients. Excellent meat and protein sources include: eggs, beef, chicken, ham, turkey, soy proteins, lean sausage, seafood, legumes, beans, and turkey. Nuts are an excellent protein source but are not always a good choice unless prepared properly. Peanut butter and other nut butters should be avoided as they are sticky and present as a choking/aspiration risk. They can however be added to foods to enhance flavor and protein. An example would be a peanut butter banana smoothie.

Meats contain varying amounts of muscle, fibers, connective tissue, fat, bone and moisture content. Most of the protein of meat is found in the muscle. Cooking meat with the bone can enhance the flavor of the meat. All bones should be removed prior to processing meat. Meat's with high fat content generally have more flavor. The tenderness of meat depends are numerous factors including age of the animal, cut of meat, heredity, diet, marbling, aging, cooking methods, and fat content. Choose meats that are lean and have a high yield of edible protein. For example, a pork chop with a large bone and large amounts of fat may not yield the proper amount of edible portion of protein. Meats can be cooked with the bone and additional fat for flavor but the trim fat and remove the bone before processing to ensure proper amounts of edible protein.

Processing meats may take a longer time than other foods. The visual appearance of meat can have a strong negative factor and affect acceptance. Poorly prepared meats can appear watering and unappealing. Meats and protein sources should have a smooth cohesive appearance like pudding or mashed potatoes.

Meats can be tough and stringy. Meats that are tough and stringy may benefit from grinding prior to adding liquid (Like broth) or sauce to the meat. Only add a small amount at a time to prevent it from becoming too thin. Only add thickeners if needed. Remember it is best to achieve a nutrient dense product. Adding too much liquid or sauce decreases the protein density and affect flavor. Very dry products puree better by adding one teaspoon of fat per serving. Fish can be dry. To improve the consistency of fish, add lemon juice, mayonnaise or tartar sauce. Adding puree sauce as a topping can enhance flavor and visual appearance.

Food molds are available to enhance the visual appearance. Scooping in a timbale form or muffin pan shape can improve appearance. Shell shaped scoops can be used. Avoid bowls and scoop dishes unless preferred for more independent eating.

Season meats and poultry with a variety of herbs and spices. Put away the salt shaker and season meats with ground herbs and spices to enhance flavor. Adding herbs and spices has many health benefits. In fact, herbs and spices contain a wide variety of antioxidants, minerals and vitamins and help maximize the nutrient density of your meals. Every time you flavor meals with herbs and spices you are literally upgrading your meal without adding a single calorie. Many herbs and spices have anti-inflammatory response when added to meals. Have plenty of ground herbs and spices available to enhance meals. Garlic powder, cinnamon, turmeric, ginger, sage, thyme, and oregano are well known for anti-inflammatory responses and go a long way toward preventing chronic illness.

Breakfast Entrees

A good breakfast is a great way to start the day. Puree yogurt or puree cottage cheese is a great way to protein into the breakfast meal. Eggs are an excellent choice of protein in the morning. Individuals who do not high cholesterol levels can enjoy an egg daily. If cholesterol is of concern, an egg white substitute is also an excellent choice since the cholesterol is in the egg yolk. Scrambled eggs are usually tolerated well in the puree diet plan and do not need further processing. For omelets, cheese can be melted on top of the egg. Vegetables in omelets should be cooked and pureed separately and added as a topping to the omelets.

Entrees

The entrée is often known as the center of plate in the food service industry. The entrée is usually the most expensive item of the meal and most people plan meals around the entrée. Beef, Chicken, Pork, Ham, Lean Sausage, Turkey, Seafood and Meatless entrée are excellent sources of protein. Ham and some sausages can contain high amounts of sodium and fat and should be used sparingly for optimal nutritional quality. Unfortunately, the protein part of the meal is usually the most rejected part of a puree diet plan even though protein is so vital. Therefore, I try and keep the entrée simple and compliment the protein source with a good sauce for flavor.

Purchasing meats and protein sources can be expensive. A great way to save money is to buy in bulk and separate into individual servings. Chicken and seafood can be purchased individually quick-frozen and the amount needed can be pulled out as needed. Smaller portions of beef, seafood and pork can be purchased from the markets with butchers. Pre-formed frozen ground beef and turkey patties can be purchased and patties pulled and prepared as needed. Purchase lean ground meat and turkey for nutrient dense protein meals. The higher fat ground meats may be lower in price but after cooking and draining the excess fat, the cost of the leaner meats per serving is less and more nutrient dense. Meats can be prepared ahead and frozen for up to 30 days and reheated before serving. For optimal flavor avoid preparing ahead and serve meats freshly made. Always reheat meats to 165 ° F.

Entrees Beef

Recipe Name: **Asian Skirt Steak**
Portion Size: 4 oz.
Servings: 1
Ingredients:
4 oz. lean skirt steak
2 tablespoons soy sauce
2 tablespoons BBQ sauce
1 teaspoon peanut butter
¼ teaspoon garlic powder
1 teaspoon cornstarch
1 teaspoon vegetable oil
Directions:
In a small bowl combine, soy sauce, BBQ sauce, peanut butter and garlic powder. Divide sauce into half. Pierce steak with fork several times. Place steak in a small zip lock bag. Pour ½ the sauce in the bag. Marinate in the refrigerator for 30 minutes. In a small pan, heat oil on medium high heat. Sauté steak turning once. Cook meats to 145 ° F. Process meat in food processor whole hot by grinding meat first and adding 1 teaspoon broth at a time until desired consistency is achieved. The meat should be smooth and consistency of mashed potatoes or pudding and not runny. For sauce, combine remaining sauce, and cornstarch. Heat in small sauce pan on medium high heat until thick and bubbly. Top puree meat with sauce.

Recipe Name: **Ground Beef Patty**
Portion Size: 4 oz.
Servings: 1
Ingredients:
3 oz. lean ground beef
dash of salt
dash of pepper
1 teaspoon minced dried onions (optional)
1/4 teaspoon ground garlic powder
2 tablespoons catsup
1 slice cheese, any type American, Cheddar, Swiss etc. (optional)
Directions:
Combine ground beef, salt, pepper, onions, and catsup in a bowl. Form into a patty. Sauté in a small pan on medium high heat. Cook meats to 165 ° F. Process meat in food processor whole hot by grinding meat first and adding 1 teaspoon broth at a time until desired consistency is achieved. The meat should be smooth and consistency of mashed potatoes or pudding and not runny. Top with cheese and melt cheese in microwave on high for 15 seconds.

Recipe Name: **Mini Meatloaf**
Portion Size: 4 oz.
Servings: 1
Ingredients:
3 oz. lean ground beef
1 egg
dash of salt
dash of pepper
2 tablespoons quick cooking oats
1 teaspoon minced dried onions
1 teaspoon prepared mustard
2 tablespoons catsup
Directions:
Combine ground beef, egg, salt, pepper, oats, onions, and mustard in a bowl. Form into a mini loaf. Bake in 350 ° for 25-30 minutes. Cook meats to 165 ° F. Process meat in food processor whole hot by grinding meat first and adding 1 teaspoon broth at a time until desired consistency is achieved. The meat should be smooth and consistency of mashed potatoes or pudding and not runny. Top with catsup.

Recipe Name: **Salisbury Steak**
Portion Size: 4 oz.
Servings: 1
Ingredients:
3 oz. lean ground beef
2 tablespoons nonfat milk
dash of salt
dash of pepper
1 teaspoon minced dried onions
1 teaspoon Worcestershire sauce
2 tablespoons bread crumbs.
For Gravy:
1 teaspoon butter or margarine
1 teaspoon all purpose flour
3 tablespoons beef broth
Directions:
Combine ground beef, milk, salt, pepper, Worcestershire sauce, onions, and breadcrumbs in a bowl. Form into a mini loaf. Bake in 350 ° for 25-30 minutes. Cook meats to 165 ° F. Process meat in food processor whole hot by grinding meat first and adding 1 teaspoon broth at a time until desired consistency is achieved. The meat should be smooth and consistency of mashed potatoes or pudding and not runny. For gravy: melt butter in small pan on medium high heat. Add flour and whisk. Stir in beef broth and cook until thick and bubbly. Top steak with gravy.

Entrees Chicken

Recipe Name: **Apple Spiced Chicken**
Portion Size: 4 oz. plus sauce
Servings: 1
Ingredients:
4 oz. boneless skinless chicken breast or thighs.
dash of salt
dash of pepper
1 teaspoon vegetable oil
 For Sauce:
2 tablespoons apple jelly
1 teaspoon lemon juice
½ teaspoon cornstarch
¼ teaspoon all spice

Directions:
In a small pan, heat oil in medium high heat. Season chicken with salt and pepper. Cook meats to 165 ° F. Process meat in food processor whole hot by grinding meat first and adding 1 teaspoon broth at a time until desired consistency is achieved. The meat should be smooth and consistency of mashed potatoes or pudding and not runny. For sauce: In a small bowl combine cornstarch, apple jelly, lemon juice, and all spice. Stir until well combined. In a small pan heat sauce until thick and bubbly. Top puree chicken with sauce while still hot.

Recipe Name: **Sauté Chicken**
Portion Size: 4 oz.
Servings: 1
Ingredients:
4 oz. boneless skinless chicken breast or thighs.
dash of salt
dash of pepper
1 teaspoon vegetable oil
Directions:
In a small pan, heat oil in medium high heat. Season chicken with salt and pepper. Cook meats to 165 ° F. Process meat in food processor whole hot by grinding meat first and adding 1 teaspoon broth at a time until desired consistency is achieved. The meat should be smooth and consistency of mashed potatoes or pudding and not runny. Top with sauce. (see variety of sauce in sauce recipe section)

Recipe Name: **Chicken with Curry Sauce**

Portion Size: 4 oz. and ½ cup sauce

Servings: 1

Ingredients:

4 oz. boneless skinless chicken breast or thighs.

dash of salt

dash of pepper

1 teaspoon vegetable oil

For Chicken Curry Sauce:

1 teaspoon vegetable oil

1 tablespoon minced onion

1 tablespoon minced green bell pepper

2 teaspoons diced pimento

¼ teaspoon garlic powder

2 tablespoons chicken broth

Dash of Worcester sauce

Dash of ginger

¼ cup plain non-fat yogurt

2 tablespoons milk (or coconut milk)

½ teaspoon curry powder

Directions:

In a small pan, heat oil in medium high heat. Season chicken with salt and pepper. Cook meats to 165 ° F. Process meat in food processor whole hot by grinding meat first and adding 1 teaspoon broth at a time until desired consistency is achieved. The meat should be smooth and consistency of mashed potatoes or pudding and not runny. For sauce, sauté onion and bell pepper in oil. Stir pimento, garlic, chicken broth, Worcester sauce, ginger, yogurt milk and curry powder. Heat through. Transfer to food processor and puree until smooth. Top chicken with sauce.

Recipe Name: **Chicken Schnitzel**
Portion Size: 4 oz.
Servings: 1
Ingredients:
4 oz. boneless skinless chicken breast or thighs.
dash of salt
dash of pepper
2 tablespoons Panko bread crumbs
1 teaspoon vegetable oil
1 teaspoon smooth Dijon mustard
1 tablespoon all purpose flour
1 tablespoon lemon juice
Directions:
In 3 separate small bowls, place flour, bread crumbs and Dijon mustard. Add 2 tablespoons water to Dijon mustard and stir. Season chicken with salt and pepper. Coat chicken with flour, then mustard then bread crumbs. In a small pan, heat oil in medium high heat. Cook meats to 165 ° F. Top with lemon juice. Process meat in food processor whole hot by grinding meat first and adding 1 teaspoon broth at a time until desired consistency is achieved. The meat should be smooth and consistency of mashed potatoes or pudding and not runny. May top with lemon sauce in sauce recipe section.

Recipe Name: **Chicken with Apple Mustard Sauce (or Pork)**
Portion Size: 4 oz. plus sauce
Servings: 1
Ingredients:
4 oz. boneless lean pork chops OR skinless chicken breast or thighs.
dash of salt
dash of pepper
1 teaspoon vegetable oil
For Sauce:
2 tablespoons apple juice
2 tablespoon apple jelly
1 tablespoon smooth Dijon mustard
½ teaspoon cornstarch
Dash of ground ginger

Directions:
In a small pan, heat oil in medium high heat. Season meat with salt and pepper. Cook meats to 165 ° F. Process meat in food processor whole hot by grinding meat first and adding 1 teaspoon broth at a time until desired consistency is achieved. The meat should be smooth and consistency of mashed potatoes or pudding and not runny. For sauce: In a small bowl combine apple jelly, apple juice, Dijon mustard and cornstarch. Stir until well combine. In a small pan heat sauce until thick and bubbly. Top puree meat with sauce while still hot.

Recipe Name: **Chicken with Apricot Ginger Teriyaki Sauce (or Pork)**
Portion Size: 4 oz. plus sauce
Servings: 1
Ingredients:
4 oz. boneless lean pork chops OR skinless chicken breast or thighs.
dash of salt
dash of pepper
1 teaspoon vegetable oil
For Sauce:
2 tablespoons apricot fruit preserves, processed until smooth
2 tablespoon soy sauce or teriyaki sauce
½ teaspoon honey
¼ teaspoon garlic powder
½ teaspoon cornstarch
Dash of ground ginger

Directions:
In a small pan, heat oil in medium high heat. Season meat with salt and pepper. Cook meats to 165 ° F. Process meat in food processor whole hot by grinding meat first and adding 1 teaspoon broth at a time until desired consistency is achieved. The meat should be smooth and consistency of mashed potatoes or pudding and not runny. For sauce: In a small bowl combine puree apricots, soy sauce, honey, ginger and cornstarch. Stir until well combine. In a small pan heat sauce until thick and bubbly. Top puree meat with sauce while still hot.

Recipe Name: **Chicken with Dijon Sauce (or Pork)**
Portion Size: 4 oz. plus sauce
Servings: 1
Ingredients:
4 oz. boneless lean pork chops OR skinless chicken breast or thighs.
dash of salt
dash of pepper
1 teaspoon vegetable oil
For Sauce:
2 tablespoons Italian Salad Dressing
¼ teaspoon onion powder
1 tablespoon smooth Dijon mustard
½ teaspoon cornstarch
Dash of ground ginger

Directions:
In a small pan, heat oil in medium high heat. Season meat with salt and pepper. Cook **meats to 165 ° F. Process meat in food processor whole hot by grinding meat first and adding 1 teaspoon broth at a time until desired consistency is achieved. The meat should be smooth and consistency of mashed potatoes or pudding and not runny. For sauce: In a small bowl combine Italian dressing, Dijon mustard, onion powder and cornstarch. Stir until well combine. In a small pan heat sauce until thick and bubbly. Top puree meat with sauce while still hot.**

Recipe Name: **Chicken with Cacciatore Sauce**
Portion Size: 4 oz. and ½ cup sauce
Servings: 1
Ingredients:
4 oz. boneless skinless chicken breast or thighs.
dash of salt
dash of pepper
1 teaspoon vegetable oil
 For Chicken Cacciatore Sauce:
1 teaspoon vegetable oil
2 tablespoons minced onion
1 tablespoon minced green bell pepper
1 tablespoon tomato paste
¼ teaspoon garlic powder
1 tablespoon chicken broth
Dash of Worcester sauce
¼ teaspoon all spice
¼ teaspoon thyme
Directions:
In a small pan, heat oil in medium high heat. Season chicken with salt and pepper. Cook meats to 165 ° F. Process meat in food processor whole hot by grinding meat first and adding 1 teaspoon broth at a time until desired consistency is achieved. The meat should be smooth and consistency of mashed potatoes or pudding and not runny. For sauce, sauté onion and bell pepper in oil. Stir in tomato paste, garlic powder, chicken broth, Worcester sauce, all spice and thyme. Heat through. Transfer to food processor and puree until smooth. Top chicken with sauce.

Recipe Name: **Chicken with Curry Mango Sauce (or Pork)**
Portion Size: 4 oz. plus sauce
Servings: 1
Ingredients:
4 oz. boneless lean pork chops OR skinless chicken breast or thighs.
dash of salt
dash of pepper
1 teaspoon vegetable oil
For Sauce:
¼ cup puree fresh or frozen mango
½ teaspoon curry
½ teaspoon cornstarch
1 tablespoon chicken broth
¼ teaspoon onion powder

Directions:
In a small pan, heat oil in medium high heat. Season meat with salt and pepper. Cook **meats to 165 ° F. Process meat in food processor whole hot by grinding meat first and adding 1 teaspoon broth at a time until desired consistency is achieved. The meat should be smooth and consistency of mashed potatoes or pudding and not runny. For sauce: In a small bowl combine puree mango, curry, chicken broth, onion powder and cornstarch. Stir until well combine. In a small pan heat sauce until thick and bubbly. Top puree meat with sauce while still hot.**

Recipe Name: **Chicken with Honey Orange Sauce (or Pork)**
Portion Size: 4 oz. plus sauce
Servings: 1
Ingredients:
4 oz. boneless lean pork chops OR skinless chicken breast or thighs.
dash of salt
dash of pepper
1 teaspoon vegetable oil
For Sauce:
2 tablespoons orange juice
2 tablespoon pineapple juice
1 tablespoon soy sauce
1 teaspoon honey
¼ teaspoon garlic powder
½ teaspoon cornstarch

Directions:
In a small pan, heat oil in medium high heat. Season meat with salt and pepper. Cook meats to 165 ° F. Process meat in food processor whole hot by grinding meat first and adding 1 teaspoon broth at a time until desired consistency is achieved. The meat should be smooth and consistency of mashed potatoes or pudding and not runny. For sauce: In a small bowl combine orange juice, pineapple juice, soy sauce, honey, garlic powder and cornstarch. Stir until well combine. In a small pan heat sauce until thick and bubbly. Top puree meat with sauce while still hot.

Recipe Name: **Chicken with Orange Mustard Sauce (or Pork)**
Portion Size: 4 oz. plus sauce
Servings: 1
Ingredients:
4 oz. boneless lean pork chops OR skinless chicken breast or thighs.
dash of salt
dash of pepper
1 teaspoon vegetable oil
For Sauce:
2 tablespoons orange juice
1 tablespoon honey
1 tablespoon smooth Dijon mustard
¼ teaspoon garlic powder
¼ teaspoon onion powder
1 teaspoon soy sauce
½ teaspoon cornstarch
Dash of ground ginger

Directions:
In a small pan, heat oil in medium high heat. Season meat with salt and pepper. Cook meats to 165 ° F. Process meat in food processor whole hot by grinding meat first and adding 1 teaspoon broth at a time until desired consistency is achieved. The meat should be smooth and consistency of mashed potatoes or pudding and not runny. For sauce: In a small bowl combine orange juice, honey, Dijon mustard, garlic powder, onion powder, soy sauce, ginger, and cornstarch. Stir until well combine. In a small pan heat sauce until thick and bubbly. Top puree meat with sauce while still hot.

Recipe Name: **Chicken with Lemon Sauce (or Pork)**
Portion Size: 4 oz. plus sauce
Servings: 1
Ingredients:
4 oz. boneless lean pork chops OR skinless chicken breast or thighs.
dash of salt
dash of pepper
1 teaspoon vegetable oil
 For Sauce:
2 tablespoons lemon juice
2 tablespoon catsup
1 tablespoon brown sugar
¼ teaspoon garlic powder
¼ teaspoon onion powder
½ teaspoon cornstarch

Directions:
In a small pan, heat oil in medium high heat. Season meat with salt and pepper. Cook meats to 165 ° F. Process meat in food processor whole hot by grinding meat first and adding 1 teaspoon broth at a time until desired consistency is achieved. The meat should be smooth and consistency of mashed potatoes or pudding and not runny. For sauce: In a small bowl combine lemon juice, catsup, brown sugar, garlic powder, onion powder and cornstarch. Stir until well combine. In a small pan heat sauce until thick and bubbly. Top puree meat with sauce while still hot.

Recipe Name: **Chicken with Spiced Peach Sauce (or Pork)**
Portion Size: 4 oz. plus sauce
Servings: 1
Ingredients:
4 oz. boneless lean pork chops OR skinless chicken breast or thighs.
dash of salt
dash of pepper
1/8 teaspoon paprika
1 teaspoon all purpose flour
1/8 teaspoon cinnamon
dash all spice
dash ground cloves
1 teaspoon vegetable oil
For Sauce:
1 teaspoon smooth Dijon mustard
1 tablespoon brown sugar
¼ teaspoon onion powder
Dash cayenne pepper
½ teaspoon cornstarch
3 tablespoons puree peaches.
Directions:
In small bowl combine, salt, pepper, paprika, flour, cinnamon, all spice, and ground cloves. Dredge meat in flour mixture. In a small pan, heat oil in medium high heat. **Cook** *meats to 165 ° F. Process meat in food processor whole hot by grinding meat first and adding 1 teaspoon broth at a time until desired consistency is achieved. The meat should be smooth and consistency of mashed potatoes or pudding and not runny. For sauce: In a small bowl combine Dijon mustard, brown sugar, onion powder, cayenne pepper, puree peaches and cornstarch. Stir until well combine. In a small pan heat sauce until thick and bubbly. Top puree meat with sauce while still hot.*

Recipe Name: **Italian Chicken**
Portion Size: 4 oz.
Servings: 1
Ingredients:
4 oz. boneless skinless chicken breast or thighs.
dash of salt
dash of pepper
1 teaspoon vegetable oil
¼ cup thick spaghetti sauce
2 tablespoons shredded mozzarella cheese
Directions:
In a small pan, heat oil in medium high heat. Season chicken with salt and pepper. Cook meats to 165 ° F. Process meat in food processor whole hot by grinding meat first and adding 1 teaspoon broth at a time until desired consistency is achieved. The meat should be smooth and consistency of mashed potatoes or pudding and not runny. Heat sauce in microwave on high for 30 seconds or until hot. Top puree chicken with sauce. Add cheese and return to microwave and heat on high until cheese is melted. (about 20 seconds)

Recipe Name: **Sesame Ginger Chicken**
Portion Size: 4 oz. plus sauce
Servings: 1
Ingredients:
4 oz. boneless skinless chicken breast or thighs
dash of salt
dash of pepper
1 teaspoon vegetable oil
For Sauce:
2 tablespoons soy sauce
1 teaspoon honey
½ teaspoon cornstarch
¼ teaspoon garlic powder
Dash of ground ginger

Directions:
In a small pan, heat oil in medium high heat. Season chicken with salt and pepper. **Cook** *meats to 165 ° F. Process meat in food processor whole hot by grinding meat first and adding 1 teaspoon broth at a time until desired consistency is achieved. The meat should be smooth and consistency of mashed potatoes or pudding and not runny. For sauce: In a small bowl combine soy sauce, honey, cornstarch, garlic powder and ginger. Stir until well combined. In a small pan heat sauce until thick and bubbly. Top puree chicken with sauce while still hot.*

Entrees Pork

Recipe Name: **Pork Chop with Chili Rub (or Chicken)**
Portion Size: 4 oz.
Servings: 1
Ingredients:
4 oz. boneless lean pork chops OR skinless chicken breast or thighs.
dash of salt
dash of pepper
¼ teaspoon garlic powder
¼ teaspoon onion powder,
1 teaspoon brown sugar,
¼ teaspoon chili powder
1 teaspoon vegetable oil
For Sauce:

Directions:
In a small bowl combine salt, pepper, garlic powder, onion powder, brown sugar, and chili powder. Rub seasoning onto meat. In a small pan, heat oil in medium high heat. Cook meats to 165 ° F. Process meat in food processor whole hot by grinding meat first and adding 1 teaspoon broth at a time until desired consistency is achieved. The meat should be smooth and consistency of mashed potatoes or pudding and not runny.

Recipe Name: **Pork Chop with Cranberry Apple Sauce (or Chicken)**

Portion Size: 4 oz. plus sauce
Servings: 1
Ingredients:
4 oz. boneless lean pork chops OR skinless chicken breast or thighs.
dash of salt
dash of pepper
1 teaspoon vegetable oil
For Sauce:
2 tablespoons jellied cranberry sauce
1 teaspoon apple juice
½ teaspoon cornstarch
2 teaspoons orange juice concentrate
Dash of ground ginger

Directions:
In a small pan, heat oil in medium high heat. Season meat with salt and pepper. Cook meats to 165 ° F. Process meat in food processor whole hot by grinding meat first and adding 1 teaspoon broth at a time until desired consistency is achieved. The meat should be smooth and consistency of mashed potatoes or pudding and not runny. For sauce: In a small bowl combine cranberry sauce, apple juice, cornstarch, orange juice concentrate and ginger. Stir until well combine. In a small pan heat sauce until thick and bubbly. Top puree meat with sauce while still hot.

Recipe Name: **Pork Chop with Apple Curry Sauce (or Chicken)**
Portion Size: 4 oz. plus sauce
Servings: 1
Ingredients:
4 oz. boneless lean pork chops OR skinless chicken breast or thighs.
dash of salt
dash of pepper
1 teaspoon vegetable oil
 For Sauce:
2 tablespoons apple juice
2 tablespoons chicken broth
1/4 teaspoon ground curry
½ teaspoon cornstarch
Dash of ground ginger

Directions:
In a small pan, heat oil in medium high heat. Season meat with salt and pepper. Cook meats to 165 ° F. Process meat in food processor whole hot by grinding meat first and adding 1 teaspoon broth at a time until desired consistency is achieved. The meat should be smooth and consistency of mashed potatoes or pudding and not runny. For sauce: In a small bowl combine chicken broth, apple juice, cornstarch, curry and ginger. Stir until well combine. In a small pan heat sauce until thick and bubbly. Top puree meat with sauce while still hot.

Recipe Name: **Pork Chop with Fresh Plum Sauce (or Chicken)**
Portion Size: 4 oz. plus sauce
Servings: 1
Ingredients:
4 oz. boneless lean pork chops OR skinless chicken breast or thighs.
dash of salt
dash of pepper
1 teaspoon vegetable oil
For Sauce:
2 tablespoons fresh plums, puree
1 tablespoon brown sugar
½ teaspoon cider vinegar
¼ teaspoon onion powder
½ teaspoon cornstarch
Dash of ground ginger

Directions:
In a small pan, heat oil in medium high heat. Season meat with salt and pepper. Cook meats to 165 ° F. Process meat in food processor whole hot by grinding meat first and adding 1 teaspoon broth at a time until desired consistency is achieved. The meat should be smooth and consistency of mashed potatoes or pudding and not runny. For sauce: In a small bowl combine puree plums, brown sugar, cider vinegar, onion powder, ginger and cornstarch. Stir until well combine. In a small pan heat sauce until thick and bubbly. Top puree meat with sauce while still hot.

Recipe Name: **Pork Chop with Honey Garlic Sauce (or Chicken)**
Portion Size: 4 oz. plus sauce
Servings: 1
Ingredients:
4 oz. boneless lean pork chops OR skinless chicken breast or thighs.
dash of salt
dash of pepper
1 teaspoon vegetable oil
For Sauce:
2 tablespoons lemon juice
1 tablespoon honey
2 tablespoon chicken broth
2 teaspoons soy sauce
½ teaspoon garlic powder
½ teaspoon cornstarch

Directions:
In a small pan, heat oil in medium high heat. Season meat with salt and pepper. Cook meats to 165 ° F. Process meat in food processor whole hot by grinding meat first and adding 1 teaspoon broth at a time until desired consistency is achieved. The meat should be smooth and consistency of mashed potatoes or pudding and not runny. For sauce: In a small bowl combine lemon juice, honey, chicken broth, soy sauce, garlic powder and cornstarch. Stir until well combine. In a small pan heat sauce until thick and bubbly. Top puree meat with sauce while still hot.

Recipe Name: **Pork Chop with Sour Cream Sauce (or Chicken)**
Portion Size: 4 oz. plus sauce
Servings: 1
Ingredients:
4 oz. boneless lean pork chops OR skinless chicken breast or thighs.
dash of salt
dash of pepper
1 teaspoon vegetable oil
For Sauce:
2 tablespoons sour cream
2 tablespoon chicken broth
¼ teaspoon paprika
¼ teaspoon garlic powder,
¼ teaspoon onion powder
Dash Worcester sauce

Directions:
In a small pan, heat oil in medium high heat. Season meat with salt and pepper. Cook meats to 165 ° F. Process meat in food processor whole hot by grinding meat first and adding 1 teaspoon broth at a time until desired consistency is achieved. The meat should be smooth and consistency of mashed potatoes or pudding and not runny. For sauce: In a small bowl combine sour cream, chicken broth, paprika, garlic powder, onion powder and Worcester sauce. Stir until well combine. In a small pan heat sauce until thick and bubbly. Top puree meat with sauce while still hot.

Entrees Seafood

Recipe Name: **Baked Cod with Lemon Dill Sauce (may use any white fish)**
Portion Size: 4 oz. plus sauce
Servings: 1
Ingredients:
**4 oz. boneless and skin less cod fillets
dash of salt
dash of pepper
dash of paprika
1 teaspoon vegetable oil
Tarter Sauce or lemon juice
 For Sauce:
2 tablespoons sour cream
1 tablespoon mayonnaise
½ teaspoon lemon juice
¼ teaspoon garlic powder
½ teaspoon dried ground dill
Dash of Worcester sauce
Salt and Pepper to taste**

Directions:
In a small pan, heat oil in medium high heat. Season fish with salt, paprika and pepper. Cook fish to 145 ° F. Process meat in food processor whole hot by grinding fish first and adding 1 teaspoon lemon juice or tarter sauce at a time until desired consistency is achieved. The fish should be smooth and consistency of mashed potatoes or pudding and not runny. For sauce: In a small bowl combine sour cream, mayonnaise. Juice, garlic powder, ground dill, and Worcester sauce. Season with salt and pepper. Top fish sauce with sauce.

Recipe Name: **Blackened Tilapia Fish (may use any white fish)**
Portion Size: 4 oz. plus sauce
Servings: 1
Ingredients:
4 oz. boneless skinless tilapia
dash of salt
dash of pepper
1/8 teaspoon paprika
1 teaspoon brown sugar,
1/8 teaspoon ground cumin
1/8 teaspoon garlic powder
1/8 teaspoon dried oregano
1 teaspoon vegetable oil
Tarter Sauce or lemon juice

Directions:
In a small bowl combine, salt, pepper, paprika, brown sugar, cumin, garlic powder, and oregano. Seasoning on fish fillet. In a small pan, heat oil in medium high heat. Cook fish to 145 ° F. Process meat in food processor whole hot by grinding fish first and adding 1 teaspoon lemon juice or tarter sauce at a time until desired consistency is achieved. The fish should be smooth and consistency of mashed potatoes or pudding and not runny. May top with lemon juice or tarter sauce.

Recipe Name: **Broiled Parmesan Fish (may use any white fish)**
Portion Size: 4 oz. plus sauce
Servings: 1
Ingredients:
4 oz. boneless skinless white fish
dash of salt
dash of pepper
2 tablespoons mayonnaise
2 tablespoons grated parmesan cheese
1/8 teaspoon grated onion
Dash of Tabasco hot pepper sauce (optional)
Tarter Sauce or lemon juice

Directions:
In a small bowl combine, mayonnaise, parmesan cheese, and grated onion. Seasoning fish fillet with salt and pepper. Place fillet in baking dish and broil for 5 minutes. Remove from oven. Spread mixture on fish. Return to broil and broil until topping is brown and food is cooked. Cook fish to 145 ° F. Process fish in food processor whole hot by grinding fish first and adding 1 teaspoon lemon juice or tarter sauce at a time until desired consistency is achieved. The fish should be smooth and consistency of mashed potatoes or pudding and not runny. Top with Tabasco sauce if desired.

Recipe Name: **Crab Cakes with Red Pepper Sauce (may also use canned tuna or salmon)**
Portion Size: 4 oz. plus sauce
Servings: 1
Ingredients:
4 oz. boneless lump crab meat, drained
2 teaspoons minced onion
1 teaspoon parsley flakes
1 teaspoon lemon juice
¼ teaspoon paprika
2 tablespoon bread crumbs
1 egg
1 teaspoon vegetable oil
Tarter Sauce or lemon juice
For Sauce:
1 tablespoon sweet red pepper, finely chopped
1 teaspoon onion, minced
1 teaspoon Dijon mustard
1 tablespoon mayonnaise
1 tablespoon sour cream
1 teaspoon lemon juice.
Dash of salt and pepper

Directions:
In a small bowl combine, crab, onion, parsley flakes, lemon juice, paprika, bread crumbs, and egg. Form into patty. In a small pan, heat oil in medium high heat. Cook patty to 145 ° F turning once. Process patty in food processor whole hot by grinding meat first and adding 1 teaspoon lemon juice or tarter sauce at a time until desired consistency is achieved. The fish should be smooth and consistency of mashed potatoes or pudding and not runny. For sauce, combine all ingredients in small food processor. Process until smooth. Top patty with sauce.

Recipe Name: **Glazed Salmon (may use any fish fillet)**
Portion Size: 4 oz. plus sauce
Servings: 1
Ingredients:
4 oz. boneless skinless salmon
1 teaspoon honey
3 tablespoons light soy sauce
1/8 teaspoon ground garlic powder
½ teaspoon cornstarch
Dash of ginger
1 teaspoon vegetable oil
Tarter Sauce or lemon juice

Directions:
In a small pan, heat oil in medium high heat. Cook fish to 145 ° F. Process meat in food processor whole hot by grinding fish first and adding 1 teaspoon lemon juice or tarter sauce at a time until desired consistency is achieved. The fish should be smooth and consistency of mashed potatoes or pudding and not runny. For glaze: combine soy sauce, honey, garlic, ginger and cornstarch. Heat in small pan until thick and bubbly. Pour over fish while still hot.

Recipe Name: **Lemon Dijon Baked Fish (may use any white fish)**
Portion Size: 4 oz. plus sauce
Servings: 1
Ingredients:
4 oz. boneless skinless white fish
dash of salt
dash of pepper
1 tablespoons Dijon mustard
2 tablespoons butter or margarine
1 teaspoon lemon juice
Dash Worchester sauce
2 tablespoons bread crumbs
Tarter Sauce or lemon juice

Directions:
In a small bowl combine, Dijon mustard, butter, lemon juice, and Worchester sauce. Seasoning fish fillet with salt and pepper. Dip fillets in mustard mixture and then bread crumbs. Bake in **350 ° F oven for 10-15 minutes** *Cook* **fish to 145 ° F. Process fish in food processor whole hot by grinding fish first and adding 1 teaspoon lemon juice or tarter sauce at a time until desired consistency is achieved. The fish should be smooth and consistency of mashed potatoes or pudding and not runny.**

Recipe Name: **Salmon Patties with Cheese Sauce (may also use canned tuna or lump crab meat) or try it with Lemon Dill Sauce**

Portion Size: 4 oz. plus sauce
Servings: 1
Ingredients:

4 oz. boneless canned salmon, drained and flaked
2 teaspoons minced onion
1 teaspoon parsley flakes
1 teaspoon lemon juice
2 tablespoon bread crumbs
1 egg
1 teaspoon Dijon mustard
1 teaspoon vegetable oil
Tarter Sauce or lemon juice
For Sauce:
2 tablespoons margarine
1 teaspoon all purpose flour
1/8 teaspoon dry mustard
2 tablespoons milk
¼ cup shredded cheese (Cheddar, Swiss or Mozzarella)
1 teaspoon onion powder
1 tablespoon mayonnaise
1 teaspoon lemon juice.
Dash of salt and pepper

Directions:
In a small bowl combine, salmon onion, parsley flakes, lemon juice, Dijon mustard, bread crumbs, and egg. Form into patty. In a small pan, heat oil in medium high heat. Cook patty to 145 ° F turning once. Process patty in food processor whole hot by grinding meat first and adding 1 teaspoon lemon juice or tarter sauce at a time until desired consistency is achieved. The fish should be smooth and consistency of mashed potatoes or pudding and not runny. For sauce, combine all ingredients in small pan. Stirring constantly, heat on low heat until well combine and cheese is melted. Top patty with sauce.

Recipe Name: **Shrimp with Marinated Chili Garlic Sauce (may also use scallops)**

Portion Size: 4 oz. p
Servings: 1
Ingredients:
4 oz. fresh shrimp, peeled, deveined and tails removed.
2 tablespoons light soy sauce
1 teaspoon chili garlic sauce
½ teaspoon minced garlic
½ teaspoon honey
1 teaspoon vegetable oil
Tarter Sauce or lemon juice

Directions:
In a small bowl combine, soy sauce, chili garlic sauce, minced garlic, and honey. Add shrimp and marinate in refrigerator for 15 minutes. Drain excess marinate and discard marinade. In a small pan, heat oil in medium high heat. Cook shrimp to 145 ° F turning. Process shrimp in food processor whole hot by grinding meat first and adding 1 teaspoon lemon juice or tarter sauce at a time until desired consistency is achieved. The fish should be smooth and consistency of mashed potatoes or pudding and not runny. For sauce, combine all ingredients in small food processor. Process until smooth.

Recipe Name: **Tuna Cakes with Creamy Citrus Sauce (may also use salmon or lump crab meat)**
Portion Size: 4 oz. plus sauce
Servings: 1
Ingredients:
4 oz. boneless canned tuna, drained and flaked
2 teaspoons minced onion
1 teaspoon red pepper, diced or pimentos
1 teaspoon lemon juice
2 tablespoon bread crumbs
1 egg
1 teaspoon vegetable oil
Tarter Sauce or lemon juice
For Sauce:
2 tablespoons sour cream
1 tablespoon mayonnaise
1/8 teaspoon lime zest
1 teaspoon lime juice
Dash of Cumin
Dash of salt and pepper

Directions:
In a small bowl combine, tuna onion, red pepper, lemon juice, bread crumbs, and egg. Form into patty. In a small pan, heat oil in medium high heat. Cook patty to 145 ° F turning once. Process patty in food processor whole hot by grinding meat first and adding 1 teaspoon lemon juice or tarter sauce at a time until desired consistency is achieved. The fish should be smooth and consistency of mashed potatoes or pudding and not runny. For sauce, combine all ingredients in small bowl. Top patty with sauce.

Entrée Turkey

Recipe Name: **Cranberry Sauced Turkey Steaks**
Portion Size: 4 oz. plus sauce
Servings: 1
Ingredients:
3 oz. lean turkey steaks
dash of salt
dash of pepper
1 tablespoon margarine, melted
1 tablespoon light soy sauce
1 tablespoon vegetable oil
For Sauce:
2 tablespoons cranberry orange sauce (canned)
1 tablespoon orange juice
½ teaspoon cornstarch
dash of cinnamon
Directions:
Combine margarine and soy sauce in a bowl. Marinate turkey steak in soy sauce for 15 minutes. Sauté turkey steak in oil in a small pan on medium high heat. Turning once. Cook meats to 165 ° F. Process meat in food processor whole hot by grinding meat first and adding 1 teaspoon broth at a time until desired consistency is achieved. The meat should be smooth and consistency of mashed potatoes or pudding and not runny. For sauce in a small saucepan stir together, cranberry orange sauce, orange juice, cornstarch and cinnamon. Cook and stir over medium heat until thickened and bubbly. Spoon sauce over puree turkey steaks.

Recipe Name: **Ground Turkey Patty (May also use beef or Chicken)**

Portion Size: 4 oz.
Servings: 1
Ingredients:
3 oz. lean ground turkey
dash of salt
dash of pepper
1 teaspoon minced dried onions
1 teaspoon parsley flakes
Dash Worcestershire sauce
1/8 teaspoon garlic powder
1 egg
Directions:
Combine ground meat, salt, pepper, egg, onions, parsley, garlic and Worcestershire sauce in a bowl. Form into a patty. Sauté in a small pan on medium high heat. Turning once. Cook meats to 165 ° F. Process meat in food processor whole hot by grinding meat first and adding 1 teaspoon broth at a time until desired consistency is achieved. The meat should be smooth and consistency of mashed potatoes or pudding and not runny. Top with your favorite sauce.

Recipe Name: **Tarragon Turkey Patty (or Chicken)**
Portion Size: 4 oz.
Servings: 1
Ingredients:
3 oz. lean ground turkey or chicken
dash of salt
dash of pepper
1 teaspoon minced dried onions
1 teaspoon parsley flakes
¼ teaspoon tarragon
¼ teaspoon dried thyme
1 teaspoon flour
1/4 teaspoon ground garlic powder
½ teaspoon smooth Dijon mustard
Sliced Cheese (optional)
Directions:
Combine ground meat, salt, pepper, onions, parsley, tarragon, thyme, garlic and mustard in a bowl. Form into a patty. Dust patty with flour. Sauté in a small pan on medium high heat. Cook meats to 165 ° F. Process meat in food processor whole hot by grinding meat first and adding 1 teaspoon broth at a time until desired consistency is achieved. The meat should be smooth and consistency of mashed potatoes or pudding and not runny. Top with cheese and melt cheese in microwave on high for 15 seconds.

Recipe Name: **Spicy Turkey Meatballs (May also use beef or Chicken)**
Portion Size: 4 oz.
Servings: 1
Ingredients:
2 oz. lean ground turkey
2 oz. spicy lean Italian sausage
dash of salt
dash of pepper
1 teaspoon minced dried onions
1/8 teaspoon garlic powder
1 egg
2 tablespoon Mozzarella cheese
Directions:
Combine ground meat, salt, pepper, onions, garlic and egg in a bowl. Form into a meatball. Sauté in a small pan on medium high heat. Cook until well browned. Cook meats to 165 ° F. Process meat in food processor whole hot by grinding meat first and adding 1 teaspoon broth at a time until desired consistency is achieved. The meat should be smooth and consistency of mashed potatoes or pudding and not runny. Form into small scoops. Top with cheese. Melt cheese in microwave for 15 seconds.

Recipe Name: **Ground Turkey with Mushroom Sauce (May also use beef or Chicken)**
Portion Size: 4 oz.
Servings: 1
Ingredients:
3 oz. lean ground turkey
dash of salt
dash of pepper
1 teaspoon minced dried onions
1 teaspoon ground thyme
1/8 teaspoon garlic powder
For Sauce:
2 tablespoons fresh mushrooms
1 tablespoon diced onion
¼ teaspoon vegetable oil
1 tablespoon broth
½ teaspoon cornstarch
Salt and Pepper to taste

Directions:
Combine ground meat, salt, pepper, onions, parsley, garlic and thyme in a bowl. Form into a patty. Sauté in a small pan on medium high heat. Turning once. Cook meats to 165 ° F. Process meat in food processor whole hot by grinding meat first and adding 1 teaspoon broth at a time until desired consistency is achieved. The meat should be smooth and consistency of mashed potatoes or pudding and not runny. For sauce, heat oil in small pan on medium high heat. Add mushroom and onions and sauté until tender. Add broth, cornstarch, and heat until thick and bubbly. Season with salt and pepper. Add to food processor and puree sauce until smooth. Top puree meat with puree mushroom sauce.

Fruits

Fruits may have a higher water content than other foods. The amount of carbohydrates and water in fruits will vary. Fruits with high water content may become watery when processed. Puree fruits should be thickened to the proper consistency if thin liquids are not tolerated. Unflavored gelatin or a thickening agent (i.e. commercial thickener, instant potato flakes, instant baby rice cereal, or xanthum gum) can be added to thicken the puree fruit. Only add the correct amount of thickening agent for the desired thickness. Adding too much thickener can affect the flavor of the fruit.

Ripeness of fruit will also affect the consistency. Fruits with tough skins should be peeled prior to processing. Seeds, pulp or tough membranes should be removed from the fruit prior to processing. Fresh fruit should be soft, ripe and peeled if the skin is tough. Most canned fruits are watery and require a stabilizer. Drain any liquid from the canned fruits prior to processing. To each ½ c. portion add 1-2 T. potato flake or another stabilizer. Pineapple, grapes, watermelon with seeds, orange, grapefruit, dried fruits and fruit skins do not process well and should be avoided. Pineapple juice and grape juice can be served and thickened to the correct thickness. Adding the zest of lemons, limes, oranges, and grapefruit can enhance the flavor of bland foods. The zest is very nutritious. Add zest to cooked cereal is a great way to enhance the flavor.

Puree bananas can turn brown over time. To avoid, serve immediately after processing or add an acid. Lemon juice works best to prevent browning. Orange will also work but not as well as it is not as acidic. If the bananas are too tart from the lemon juice a small amount of sugar (1/2 teaspoon per ½ cup) can be added.

Salad Dressing

Home made salad dressing can be added to vegetables, fruits or green salads to enhance the flavor. Choose your favorite dressing and top puree vegetables, fruits or green salads. Salad dressing can be made ahead and kept in the refrigerator for 1 week.

Recipe Name: **Asian Ginger Dressing**
Portion Size: 1 cup
Servings: 1 = 2 tablespoons
Ingredients:
3 cloves garlic
2 tablespoons minced fresh ginger or 1 teaspoon ground ginger
¾ cup olive oil
½ cup soy sauce
3 tablespoons honey
¼ cup water
Directions:
In a food processor, combine all the ingredients. Blend until smooth

Recipe Name: **Avocado Cilantro Dressing**
Portion Size: 2 cups
Servings: 1 = 2 tablespoons
Ingredients:
1 large ripe avocado
1 teaspoon salt
3 lemons juiced
1 cup light mayonnaise
3 tablespoons Cilantro
1/4 cup olive oil
¼ teaspoon pepper
Directions:
In a food processor, combine all the ingredients. Blend until smooth

Recipe Name: **Balsamic Honey Mustard Dressing**
Portion Size: 1 cup
Servings: 1 = 2 tablespoons
Ingredients:
2 cloves garlic
¼ cup honey
¼ teaspoon salt
¼ cup Dijon mustard
1/2 cup olive oil
¾ cup balsamic vinegar
¼ teaspoon pepper
Directions:
In a food processor, combine all the ingredients. Blend until smooth

Recipe Name: **Basil and Garlic Vinaigrette Dressing**
Portion Size: 1 cup
Servings: 1 = 2 tablespoons
Ingredients:
3 cloves garlic
½ cup fresh chopped basil
2/3 cup olive oil
1/3 cup balsamic vinegar
¼ teaspoon pepper
¼ teaspoon salt
1/2 cup olive oil
Directions:
In a food processor, combine all the ingredients. Blend until smooth

Recipe Name: **Blue Cheese Dressing**
Portion Size: 2 1/2 cups
Servings: 1 = 2 tablespoons
Ingredients:
1 1/3 light mayonnaise
¾ cup light sour cream
1 teaspoon Worcestershire sauce
½ teaspoon dry mustard
2 cloves garlic
4 oz. blue cheese crumbled
½ teaspoon salt
½ teaspoon ground black pepper
Directions:
In a food processor, combine all the ingredients. Blend until smooth

Recipe Name: **Buttermilk Dressing**
Portion Size: 2 cups
Servings: 1 = 2 tablespoons
Ingredients:
½ cup light mayonnaise
½ cup light sour cream
1 cup buttermilk
1 teaspoon dried oregano
1 teaspoon garlic powder
1 tablespoon dried chives
1 tablespoon dried parley
1 teaspoon dried dill
½ teaspoon ground black pepper
2 tablespoons Parmesan cheese
Directions:
In a food processor, combine all the ingredients. Blend until smooth

Recipe Name: **Carrot and Ginger Dressing**
Portion Size: 1 3/4 cups
Servings: 1 = 2 tablespoons
Ingredients:
1 teaspoon ground ginger
3 medium carrots, soften in the microwave
¼ cup rice vinegar
1 tablespoon soy sauce
1 tablespoon Asian Sesame oil
¼ teaspoon salt
½ cup vegetable oil
¼ cup water
Directions:
In a food processor, combine all the ingredients. Blend until smooth

Recipe Name: **Citrus Dressing**
Portion Size: 1 3/4 cups
Servings: 1 = 2 tablespoons
Ingredients:
½ cup white balsamic vinegar
1 tablespoon orange juice
1 tablespoon grapefruit juice
1 tablespoon fresh lime juice
1 tablespoon fresh lemon juice
¼ cup olive oil
¼ cup grated Romano cheese
¼ teaspoon salt
¼ teaspoon pepper
Directions:
In a food processor, combine all the ingredients. Blend until smooth

Recipe Name: **Citrus Parmesan Dressing**
Portion Size: 1 3/4 cups
Servings: 1 = 2 tablespoons
Ingredients:
1/3 cup grated Parmesan cheese
zest and juice of 2 oranges
2 tablespoons minced red onions.
¼ cup white wine vinegar
1/2 cup olive oil
¼ teaspoon salt
¼ teaspoon pepper
Directions:
In a food processor, combine all the ingredients. Blend until smooth.

Recipe Name: **Creamy Basil Dressing**
Portion Size: 3 cups
Servings: 1 = 2 tablespoons
Ingredients:
½ cup light mayonnaise
½ cup minced onions
½ cup chopped fresh basil or 2 tablespoons dried
zest and juice of 2 lemons
¼ teaspoon salt
¼ teaspoon pepper
1 cup light sour cream
Directions:
In a food processor, combine all the ingredients. Blend until smooth.

Recipe Name: **Creamy Italian Dressing**
Portion Size: 1 cup
Servings: 1 = 2 tablespoons
Ingredients:
½ cup light mayonnaise
1/3 cup white wine vinegar
1 teaspoon vegetable oil
2 tablespoon honey
2 tablespoons Parmesan cheese
2 tablespoons Romano cheese
2 cloves garlic, minced
½ teaspoon Italian seasoning
½ teaspoon dried parsley
1 tablespoon lemon juice
Directions:
In a food processor, combine all the ingredients. Blend until smooth.

Recipe Name: **Creamy Lemon Garlic Dressing**
Portion Size: 2 ¾ cups
Servings: 1 = 2 tablespoons
Ingredients:
¾ cup light mayonnaise
2 fresh squeezed lemons, plus zest
2 garlic cloves, minced
½ teaspoon salt
1 cup milk
1 cup Parmesan cheese, grated
Directions:
In a food processor, combine all the ingredients. Blend until smooth.

Recipe Name: **Lemon Dijon Vinaigrette Dressing**
Portion Size: 1 cup
Servings: 1 = 2 tablespoons
Ingredients:
1 tablespoon Dijon mustard
¼ cup olive oil
1/3 cup lemon juice
1 teaspoon honey
¼ teaspoon salt
¼ teaspoon pepper
Directions:
In a food processor, combine all the ingredients. Blend until smooth.

Recipe Name: **Dill Dressing (great on fish)**
Portion Size: 3 cups
Servings: 1 = 2 tablespoons
Ingredients:
1 cup nonfat plain yogurt
2 lemons, juiced plus zest
3 tablespoons red onion, minced
2 tablespoons parsley flakes
¼ teaspoon salt
¼ teaspoon pepper
1 tablespoon dried dill
Directions:
In a food processor, combine all the ingredients. Blend until smooth.

Recipe Name: **French Dressing**
Portion Size: 1/3 cups
Servings: 1 = 2 tablespoons
Ingredients:
1/3 cup wine or cider vinegar
1 cup olive or vegetable oil
½ cup minced onions
lemons
¼ teaspoon salt
¼ teaspoon pepper
Directions:
In a food processor, combine all the ingredients. Blend until smooth.

Recipe Name: **Greek Dressing**
Portion Size: 1 1/3 cups
Servings: 1 = 2 tablespoons
Ingredients:
3 cloves garlic, minced
1 teaspoon dried oregano
1 teaspoon dried basil
1 teaspoon onion powder
2 tablespoons creamy Dijon style mustard
1 cup red wine vinegar
1/3 cup olive oil
¼ teaspoon salt
¼ teaspoon pepper
Directions:
In a food processor, combine all the ingredients. Blend until smooth.

Recipe Name: **Honey Mustard Salad Dressing**
Portion Size: 3 cups
Servings: 1 = 2 tablespoons
Ingredients:
1 cup light mayonnaise
2 tablespoons minced red onions
2 tablespoons creamy Dijon mustard
¼ cup honey
1 teaspoon parsley flakes
¼ teaspoon salt
¼ teaspoon pepper
1/3 cup oil
Directions:
In a food processor, combine all the ingredients. Blend until smooth.

Recipe Name: **Ranch Buttermilk Dressing**
Portion Size: 1 cup
Servings: 1 = 2 tablespoons
Ingredients:
2 cloves garlic, minced
2 tablespoons minced onions
1 tablespoon parsley flakes or cilantro flakes
2 tablespoons lime juice
¼ teaspoon salt
¼ teaspoon pepper
¾ cup buttermilk
Directions:
In a food processor, combine all the ingredients. Blend until smooth.

Recipe Name: **Southwestern Salad Dressing**
Portion Size: ¾ cup
Servings: 1 = 2 tablespoons
Ingredients:
½ cup Ranch style salad dressing
¼ cup honey barbecue sauce
Directions:
In a food processor, combine all the ingredients. Blend until smooth.

Recipe Name: **Sweet and Sour Oriental Dressing**
Portion Size: 1 cup
Servings: 1 = 2 tablespoons
Ingredients:
¼ cup plum sauce
¼ cup rice wine vinegar
1 clove garlic, minced
1/3 cup peanut oil
1 *Directions:*
In a food processor, combine all the ingredients. Blend until smooth.

Recipe Name: **Sweet Dijon Dressing**
Portion Size: 3/4 cup
Servings: 1 = 2 tablespoons
Ingredients:
¼ cup olive oil
2 teaspoons sugar
¼ cup apple cider vinegar
¼ cup Dijon mustard
¼ teaspoon salt
¼ teaspoon pepper
Directions:
In a food processor, combine all the ingredients. Blend until smooth.

Recipe Name: **Tangy Basil Vinaigrette Dressing**
Portion Size: 1 ½ cups
Servings: 1 = 2 tablespoons
Ingredients:
2 cloves garlic, minced
½ cup olive oil
¼ cup honey
½ cup apple cider vinegar
¼ cup Dijon mustard
2 tablespoons dried basil, or ¼ cup minced fresh
¼ teaspoon salt
¼ teaspoon pepper
Directions:
In a food processor, combine all the ingredients. Blend until smoot.

Recipe Name: **Tangy Lime Dressing**
Portion Size: 1 cup
Servings: 1 = 2 tablespoons
Ingredients:
Juice of 3 small fresh limes (plus zest) or ¼ cup lime juice
2 tablespoons olive oil
2 tablespoons honey
2 tablespoons rice vinegar
2 teaspoons Dijon mustard
2 cloves fresh garlic, minced or ½ teaspoon garlic powder
2 Tablespoons fresh cilantro, minced or 1 teaspoon dried.
¼ teaspoon salt
¼ teaspoon pepper
Directions:
In a food processor, combine all the ingredients. Blend until smooth

Recipe Name: **Thousand Island Dressing**
Portion Size: 2 1/2 cups
Servings: 1 = 2 tablespoons
Ingredients:
1 cup light mayonnaise

¼ teaspoon salt
¼ teaspoon pepper
½ cup ketchup
1/2 cup sweet pickle relish
Directions:
In a food processor, combine all the ingredients. Blend until smooth

Sauces

Sauces are an excellent way to add flavor, moisture and visual appeal to another dish. The sauce can maximize flavor or jazz up any meal. Homemade sauce is a delicious way to enhance a meal. Sauces can be added to meats, poultry, fish, starches (like rice or pasta), fruits, desserts or vegetables. To maximize flavor visual appeal, use the sauce as a topping rather than blending in with the food. Most homemade sauces can be keep in the refrigerator for 5-7 days.

Recipe Name: **Aioli Garlic Sauce**
Portion Size: 1 cup
Servings: 1 = 2 tablespoons
Ingredients:
¾ cup light mayonnaise
3 cloves garlic, minced
1 tablespoon lemon juice
¼ teaspoon salt
¼ teaspoon ground pepper
Directions:

In a food processor, combine all the ingredients. Blend until smooth.

Recipe Name: **Alfredo Sauce**
Portion Size: 2 cups
Servings: 1 = ¼ cup
Ingredients:
¼ cup butter
1 (8oz.) light cream cheese
1 teaspoon garlic powder
2 cups milk
6 oz. grated Parmesan cheese
¼ teaspoon ground pepper
Directions:
In a large saucepan oil over medium heat, melt butter. Add cream cheese and garlic powder, stirring constantly with wire whisk until smooth. Slowly pour in milk and whisk. Stir in Parmesan cheese and pepper. Bring to a boil, reduce heat and simmer for 20 minutes. Serve hot.

Recipe Name: **Apple Yogurt Sauce (great on fruit)**
Portion Size: 1 ¼ cup
Servings: 1 = 2 tablespoons
Ingredients:
¼ cup applesauce
1 cup vanilla yogurt
¼ teaspoon cinnamon
Directions:

 In a food processor, combine all the ingredients. Blend until smooth.

Recipe Name: **Basil Aioli Sauce**
Portion Size: 1 cup
Servings: 1 = 2 tablespoons
Ingredients:
1/2 cup light mayonnaise
1 clove garlic, minced
1 teaspoon lemon juice
2 tablespoons olive oil
½ cup lightly packed fresh basil, washed and trimmed
¼ teaspoon salt
Dash of hot pepper sauce (optional)
Directions:

 In a food processor, combine all the ingredients. Blend until smooth.

Recipe Name: **Basil Sauce**
Portion Size: 1 cup
Servings: 1 = 2 tablespoons
Ingredients:
1/2 cup light mayonnaise
1 tablespoon onion, minced
1 clove garlic, minced

½ cup sour cream
1/4 cup lightly packed fresh basil, washed and trimmed or 2 teaspoons dried
¼ teaspoon salt
¼ teaspoon Worcestershire sauce
¼ teaspoon ground pepper

Directions:

In a food processor, combine all the ingredients. Blend until smooth.

Recipe Name: **Blueberry Sauce- (Great on puree cakes, breads, or fruits)**
Alternate: Blackberry sauce, Raspberry Sauce, Mango Sauce, Cherry Sauce or Peach Sauce
Portion Size: 1 1/2 cup
Servings: 1 = 2 tablespoons
Ingredients:

1 cup fresh or frozen blueberries (* or other fresh or frozen fruit: Apricots, Blackberries, Raspberries, Mangos, Cherries or Peaches)
½ cup orange juice
1/3 cup sugar
¼ cup cold water
2 tablespoons cornstarch
Directions:

In a medium sauce pan over medium heat, combine blueberries (or other fruit), 2 tablespoons cup of water, orange juice and sugar. Stir gently and bring to boil. In a cup or small bowl. Mix together the cornstarch and 2 tablespoons cup cold water. Gently stir the cornstarch into the fruit. Simmer 3 to 4 minutes. Remove from heat. In a food processor, combine all the ingredients. Blend until smooth. Serve warm or chill and serve cold.

Recipe Name: **Chili Garlic Sauce**
Portion Size: 1/2 cup
Servings: 1 = 2 tablespoons
Ingredients:
1/2 cup light mayonnaise
1 teaspoon sugar
2 teaspoons chili garlic sauce
Directions:

 In a food processor, combine all the ingredients. Blend until smooth. Chill.

Recipe Name: **Chipotle Sauce**
Portion Size: 1 cup
Servings: 1 = 2 tablespoons
Ingredients:
1/2 cup light mayonnaise
½ cup plain yogurt
2 teaspoons pureed chipotle peppers in adobo sauce
Directions:

 In a food processor, combine all the ingredients. Blend until smooth. Chill.

Recipe Name: **Avocado Cilantro Sauce**
Portion Size: 1 cup
Servings: 1 = 2 tablespoons
Ingredients:
1 avocado, peeled, seed removed and diced
1 clove garlic, minced
1 teaspoon lemon or lime juice
1 teaspoon olive oil
¼ teaspoon salt
¼ teaspoon ground pepper
½ cup plain low-fat yogurt
Directions:

 In a food processor, combine all the ingredients. Blend until smooth. Serve immediately. Store in refrigerator for no more than 24 hours.

Recipe Name: **Cranberry Mustard Sauce**
Portion Size: 1 cup
Servings: 1 = 2 tablespoons
Ingredients:
1 can (14 oz..) jellied cranberry sauce
3 tablespoons Dijon Mustard
2 tablespoons brown sugar
Directions:

In a food processor, combine all the ingredients. Blend until smooth.

Recipe Name: **Creamy Cantaloupe Sauce** Good for moistening dry food items like cakes, cookies or breads (Or use Apricots, Blueberries, Raspberries, Strawberries, Peaches, Pears, Mango, Bananas)

Portion Size: 1 cup
Servings: 1 = 2 tablespoons
Ingredients:
1/2 cup yogurt
1 cup cubed cantaloupe (or other fruit)
4 teaspoons sugar or honey
Directions:

Wash, peel, trim and remove seeds from fruit. In a food processor, combine all the ingredients. Blend until smooth.

Recipe Name: **Creamy Dill Sauce**
Portion Size: 2/3 cup
Servings: 1 = 2 tablespoons
Ingredients:
1/3 cup mayonnaise
1/3 cup sour cream
2 teaspoons dried dill
¼ teaspoon garlic powder
1 teaspoon lemon juice
¼ teaspoon salt
¼ teaspoon ground pepper
Directions:

In a food processor, combine all the ingredients. Blend until smooth.

Recipe Name: **Creamy Paprika Sauce**
Portion Size: 1 cup
Servings: 1 = 2 tablespoons
Ingredients:
1/4 cup mayonnaise
1/3 cup sour cream
1 tablespoon paprika
¼ cup milk
¼ teaspoon garlic powder
1 teaspoon Worcestershire sauce
¼ teaspoon salt
¼ teaspoon ground pepper
Directions:

 In a food processor, combine all the ingredients. Blend until smooth.

Recipe Name: **Creamy Parmesan Garlic Sauce**
Portion Size: 1 cup
Servings: 1 = 2 tablespoons
Ingredients:
½ cup grated Parmesan Cheese
¼ cup milk
4 oz. cream cheese
3 cloves garlic, minced
1 teaspoon parsley flakes
¼ teaspoon salt
¼ teaspoon ground pepper
Directions:

 In a food processor, combine all the ingredients. Blend until smooth.

Recipe Name: **Creamy Tomato Basil Sauce**
Great on Puree Pasta
Portion Size: 1 cup
Servings: 1 = ¼ cup
Ingredients:
2 tablespoons grated Parmesan Cheese
2 tablespoons butter
¼ cup milk
4 oz. cream cheese
3 cloves garlic, minced or 1 teaspoon ground garlic
2 teaspoons dried basil flakes
¼ teaspoon salt
¼ teaspoon ground pepper
½ cup tomato sauce
½ teaspoon sugar
Directions:

In a large saucepan oil over medium heat, melt butter. Add cream cheese and garlic powder, stirring constantly with wire whisk until smooth. Slowly pour in milk and whisk. Stir in Parmesan cheese, basil, sugar, and pepper. Bring to a boil, reduce heat and simmer for 5 minutes. Slowly stir in tomato sauce and heat through. Serve hot.

Recipe Name: **Curry Sauce (good on meats or steamed puree vegetables)**
Portion Size: 1 cup
Servings: 1 = 2 tablespoons
Ingredients:
½ teaspoon olive oil
2 tablespoons onion, minces
1 clove garlic, minced
¼ teaspoon ground cinnamon
¼ teaspoon ground black pepper
¼ teaspoon ground coriander
½ teaspoon ground cumin
¼ teaspoon ground turmeric
Dash of Cayenne pepper (optional)
1 small tomato, washed, trimmed and chopped
1 tablespoon dried cilantro
¾ cup plain yogurt
1 teaspoon lemon juice
Directions:

In a food processor, combine all the ingredients. Blend until smooth. In a sauce pan, add all ingredients. Bring to boil, reduce heat and simmer for 3 to 5 minutes. Serve warm.

Recipe Name: **Feta Yogurt Sauce**
Portion Size: 1 ½ cup
Servings: 1 = 2 tablespoons
Ingredients:
1 cup plain Greek yogurt
1 small cucumber, washed, peeled, seeds removed, chopped
1 clove garlic, minced
1 tablespoon dried mint or parsley
½ cup (2oz.) crumbled feta cheese
1 teaspoon lemon juice
¼ teaspoon salt
¼ teaspoon ground pepper
Directions:

In a food processor, combine all the ingredients. Blend until smooth.

Recipe Name: **Garlic Curry Sauce**
Portion Size: 1 cup
Servings: 1 = 2 tablespoons
Ingredients:
1/2 cup mayonnaise
2 teaspoons curry powder
½ cup plain yogurt
1 clove garlic, minced
1 tablespoon ketchup
2 tablespoon onions, minced
¼ teaspoon ground ginger
½ teaspoon chili powder
¼ teaspoon salt
¼ teaspoon ground pepper
1 tablespoon olive oil
Directions:

In a food processor, combine all the ingredients. Blend until smooth. Chill.

Recipe Name: **Honey Mustard Sauce**
Portion Size: 1 cup
Servings: 1 = 2 tablespoons
Ingredients:
2/3 cup mayonnaise
2 tablespoons Dijon mustard
2 tablespoons prepared yellow mustard
2 teaspoons lemon juice
2 tablespoons honey
Directions:

In a food processor, combine all the ingredients. Blend until smooth.

Recipe Name: **Hot Fudge Sauce**
Portion Size: 1 3/4 cup
Servings: 1 = 2 tablespoons
Ingredients:
1/3 cup mayonnaise
¾ cup granulated sugar
½ cup cocoa
½ cup plus 2 tablespoons evaporated milk (5 oz. can)
1/3 cup light corn syrup
1/3 cup margarine
1 teaspoon vanilla
Directions:

In small saucepan combine sugar and cocoa; blend in evaporated milk and corn syrup. Cook over medium heat, stirring constantly, until mixture boils; boil and stir margarine and vanilla. Serve warm. Makes about 1 3/4 cups sauce

Recipe Name: **Lemon Dill Yogurt Sauce**
Portion Size: 1 cup
Servings: 1 = 2 tablespoons
Ingredients:
1 cup plain yogurt
2 clove garlic, minced
1 tablespoon dried dill
1 teaspoon lemon juice
¼ teaspoon salt
¼ teaspoon ground pepper
Directions:

In a food processor, combine all the ingredients. Blend until smooth.

Recipe Name: **Marinara Sauce**
Portion Size: 2 cups
Servings: 1 = ¼ cup
Ingredients:
2 cups crushed tomatoes
2 teaspoons dried basil
1 teaspoon oregano
1 tablespoon olive oil
¼ cup onion, minced
2 cloves garlic, minced
¼ teaspoon salt
¼ teaspoon ground pepper
½ teaspoon sugar
Directions:

In a large saucepan oil over medium heat. Sauté onion and garlic until onions are clear. Stir in tomatoes, basil, oregano, salt, pepper, and sugar. Bring to a boil, reduce heat and simmer for 20 minutes. Serve warm.

Recipe Name: **Mexican sauce**
Portion Size: 1 cup
Servings: 1 = 2 tablespoons
Ingredients:
1/3 cup tomato sauce
¼ cup water
1 tablespoon dried cilantro
2 tablespoons onion, minced
1 clove garlic, minced
2 tablespoons brown sugar
1 tablespoon lemon juice
1 teaspoon oil
1 teaspoon Worcestershire sauce
1 tablespoon chili powder
¼ teaspoon ground cumin
¼ teaspoon salt
¼ teaspoon ground pepper
Directions:

In a food processor, combine all the ingredients. Blend until smooth. Serve warm or at room temperature.

Recipe Name: **Mushroom Sauce**
Portion Size: 1 cups
Servings: 1 = 2 tablespoons
Ingredients:
2 tablespoons milk
1 tablespoon cornstarch
½ cup beef or chicken broth
1 tablespoon olive oil
1 ½ cups fresh white mushrooms. Washed, trimmed and sliced
¼ cup onion, chopped

Directions:

In a small bowl, combine milk and cornstarch; set aside. In a small skillet, heat oil over high heat. Add mushrooms and onion; cook and stir over moderate heat until mushrooms and golden, about 10 minutes. Stir in broth; bring to a boil. Stir cornstarch mixture into mushroom mixture in skillet. Cook over high heat, stirring constantly, until slightly thickened, about 1 minute in a food processor, combine all the ingredients. Blend until smooth. Serve warm.

Recipe Name: **Orange Dipping Sauce**
Portion Size: 1 cup
Servings: 1 = 2 tablespoons
Ingredients:
½ cup orange marmalade
¼ cup honey
¼ cup Dijon mustard
hot pepper sauce to taste (optional)
Directions:

In a food processor, combine all the ingredients. Blend until smooth. Serve immediately, or refrigerate in a covered container. Serve hot or cold.

Recipe Name: **Pan Gravy**
Portion Size: 1 cup
Servings: 1 = 2 tablespoons
Ingredients:
1 teaspoon dripping from roast or poultry (if available)
2 tablespoons flour
2 tablespoons oil
¾ cup chicken or beef broth
Dash Worcestershire sauce (optional)
¼ teaspoon salt
¼ teaspoon ground pepper
Directions:

In a small pan heat oil over medium high heat. Add oil and stir to coast. Add broth and stir. Stirring frequently, bring to boil. Reduce heat and simmer thick and bubbly. Serve hot.

Recipe Name: **Peach and Ginger Sauce**
Portion Size: 1 cup
Servings: 1 = 2 tablespoons
Ingredients:
1 cup canned diced peaches, drained
1 teaspoon oil
1 tablespoon onion, minced
½ teaspoon ground ginger
1 clove garlic, minced
¼ teaspoon ground cinnamon
1/4 teaspoon yellow mustard powder
¼ teaspoon salt
¼ teaspoon ground pepper
1 tablespoon cornstarch
Directions:

In a small pan, heat oil to medium high heat. Add onions and garlic. Sauté until tender. Add peaches, ginger, brown sugar, cinnamon, mustard, cornstarch and salt. Bring to boil. Reduce heat and simmer for 10 minutes, stirring occasionally in a food processor, combine all the ingredients. Blend until smooth. Serve warm.

Recipe Name: **Peanut Sauce**
Portion Size: 1 cup
Servings: 1 = 2 tablespoons
Ingredients:
½ cup natural style creamy peanut butter
2 tablespoons water
1 tablespoon Hoisin sauce
1 tablespoon lime juice
2 teaspoons soy sauce
1 teaspoon sugar
1 teaspoon garlic chili paste (found in Asian section of market)
1 clove garlic, minced
½ teaspoon sesame oil
Directions:

In a food processor, combine all the ingredients. Blend until smooth. Serve at room temperature or warm.

Recipe Name: **Pesto Sauce**
Portion Size: 1 1/2 cup
Servings: 1 = 2 tablespoons
Ingredients:
1 cup Fresh Basil
¼ cup Parmesan cheese
¼ cup Pine nuts
2 cloves garlic, minced
¼ teaspoon salt
¼ teaspoon ground pepper
1 tablespoon olive oil

Directions:

In a food processor, combine all the ingredients. Blend until smooth. Serve warm, cold or at room temperature.

Recipe Name: **Plum Sauce**
Portion Size: 1 cup
Servings: 1 = 2 tablespoons
Ingredients:
¾ cup plum jam
2 tablespoons vinegar
1 tablespoon brown sugar
1 tablespoon onion, minced
½ teaspoon ground ginger
Dash red pepper sauce (optional)
Directions:

In a medium saucepan over medium heat, combine jam vinegar, brown sugar, dried onion, red pepper sauce, garlic and ginger. Bring to a boil, stirring. Remove from heat. In a food processor, combine all the ingredients. Blend until smooth. Chill in refrigerator for 30 minutes. Serve

Recipe Name: **Seafood Sauce**
Portion Size: 1 cup
Servings: 1 = 2 tablespoons
Ingredients:
½ cup mayonnaise
2 tablespoon chili sauce
1 teaspoon creole mustard (optional)
Dash Louisiana –style hot sauce (optional)
1 tablespoon lemon juice
½ teaspoon Worcestershire sauce
2 tablespoons, onion, minced
1 cloves garlic, minced
1 teaspoon parsley flakes
¼ teaspoon chili powder
¼ teaspoon salt
¼ teaspoon ground pepper
1 tablespoon olive oil

Directions:

In a food processor, combine all the ingredients. Blend until smooth. Chill for 20 minutes.

Recipe Name: **Spicy Mango Sauce**
Portion Size: 1 cup
Servings: 1 = 2 tablespoons
Ingredients:
3/4 cup Fresh or frozen mango, finely chopped
¼ cup rice vinegar
1 teaspoon lime juice
Dash cayenne pepper (optional)
1 cloves garlic, mined
¼ teaspoon salt
¼ teaspoon ground pepper
½ teaspoon hot chili paste
1 tablespoon fresh cilantro or 1 teaspoon dried

Directions:

In a food processor, combine all the ingredients. Blend until smooth. Chill

Recipe Name: **Tahini Yogurt Sauce**
Portion Size: 1 1/4 cup
Servings: 1 = 2 tablespoons
Ingredients:
1 cup plain Greek yogurt
3 tablespoon tahini sauce
2 tablespoons lemon juice
2 cloves garlic, mined

Directions:

In a food processor, combine all the ingredients. Blend until smooth. Serve warm, cold or at room temperature.

Recipe Name: **Tartar Sauce**
Portion Size: 1 1/2 cup
Servings: 1 = 2 tablespoons
Ingredients:
1 cup mayonnaise
2 teaspoons sweet pickle relish
1 teaspoon yellow mustard
1 teaspoon lemon juice
¼ teaspoon ground pepper

Directions:

In a food processor, combine all the ingredients. Blend until smooth. Chill.

Recipe Name: **Teriyaki Sauce**
Portion Size: 2 cups
Servings: 1 = 2 tablespoons
Ingredients:
2/3 cup mirin (Japanese sweet rice wine)
1 cup soy sauce
4 teaspoons rice vinegar
1 teaspoon sesame oil
1/3 cup sugar
7 cloves garlic, mined
¼ teaspoon ground pepper
1 teaspoon ground ginger (or 1 tablespoon fresh ginger, minced)
Directions:

Bring mirin to a boil in a saucepan over high heat. Reduce heat to medium-low, and simmer for 10 minutes. Pour in soy sauce, rice vinegar, sesame oil, and sugar. Season with garlic, ginger, pepper flakes, and black pepper; simmer an additional 5 minutes. Store in a tightly sealed container in the refrigerator

Soups

Soups can be a great way to increase your vegetable intake. Soups can be very comforting especially on cold days. Homemade soups are a great choice to control the amount of salt in the diet. Canned soups can have a lot of salt. Thin soups should be thickened to correct consistency if thin liquids are not tolerated.

Recipe Name: **Baked Acorn Squash Soup**
(or can be made with other winter squashes like; Butternut Squash, Kaboca, Hubbard, Delicata, Blue Hokkaido, Pumpkin)
Portion Size: 1 1/4 cup
Servings: 1 = 1 cup
Ingredients:
1 Acorn squash, washed, halved and seeds removed.
1 tablespoon olive oil
2 tablespoons brown sugar
Salt and pepper to taste
¼ teaspoon ground cinnamon
2 tablespoons evaporated milk
Directions:

Preheat oven to 350 degrees. Place squash in a shallow baking pan, cut side down. Bake in preheated oven for 30 minutes. Turn cut side up; Season with salt and pepper, dot with butter and sprinkle with brown sugar and cinnamon. Bake for 20 minutes or until tender. Remove and peel squash in a food processor, combine all the ingredients. Blend until smooth. Add evaporated milk and heat through.

Recipe Name: **Black Bean Soup**
Portion Size: 1 1/4 cup
Servings: 1 = 1 cup
Ingredients:
1 tablespoon olive oil
2 tablespoons onion, chopped
2 tablespoons green bell pepper, chopped
1 small can (8oz.) black beans, drained and rinsed
2 tablespoons carrot, peeled and chopped
¼ cup chicken broth
¼ teaspoon cumin
¼ teaspoon garlic powder
¼ teaspoon ground black pepper
2 tablespoons sour cream

Directions:

Wash and prepare onions, green pepper and carrots. Heat the oil in a small pot over medium heat. Stir in the onion, bell pepper, carrot, and garlic, and cook 5 minutes, until tender. In a food processor add vegetables, beans and broth puree until smooth. Return to pot and bring to boil. Mix in cumin and black pepper. Simmer 5 minutes. Garnish with sour cream.

Recipe Name: **Black Eye Peas Soup**
Portion Size: 1 1/4 cup
Servings: 1 = 1 cup
Ingredients:
1 tablespoon olive oil
2 tablespoons onion, chopped
2 tablespoons diced tomatoes
1 small can (8oz.) black eyed peas, drained and rinsed
2 tablespoons carrot, peeled and chopped
2 tablespoons celery
¼ cup beef broth
1 teaspoon dried basil

Directions:

Wash and prepare onions, celery, and carrots. Heat the oil in a small pot over medium heat. Stir in the onion, celery, carrot, and tomatoes and cook 5 minutes, until tender. In a food processor, vegetables, black eyed peas, basil, and broth until smooth. Return to pot and bring to boil. Simmer 5 minutes.

Recipe Name: **Carrot Ginger Soup**
Portion Size: 1   cup
Servings: 1 = 1 cup
Ingredients:
1 teaspoon olive oil
2 large carrots, washed, peeled and diced
2 tablespoons onion, chopped
¼ teaspoon ground black pepper
2 tablespoons plain Greek yogurt
2 tablespoons chicken broth
¼ teaspoon ground ginger
Directions:

Wash and prepare onions, and carrots. Heat the oil in a small pot over medium heat. Stir in the onion, celery, carrot, cook 5 minutes, until tender. Add chicken broth and heat through. Transfer to food processor, and puree until smooth. Return to pot and bring to boil. Simmer 5 minutes.
Top with yogurt

Recipe Name: **Cream *of* Carrot Soup**
This is a base for any cream of vegetable soup. Substitute these other vegetables for carrots to make a variety of soups: Asparagus, Beets, Poblano or Bell Peppers, Cauliflower, Celery, Spinach, Kale, Parsnips, Mushrooms, or Cabbage
Portion Size: 1 cup
Servings: 1 = 1 cup
Ingredients:

1 teaspoon olive oil
2 large carrots, washed, peeled and diced (1/2 cup other vegetable)
2 tablespoons onion, chopped
2 tablespoons celery, chopped
2 tablespoons potatoes, peeled and chopped
½ teaspoon parsley flakes
¼ cup chicken broth
¼ cup evaporated milk or half and half
salt and pepper to taste.
Directions:

Wash and prepare vegetables. Heat the oil in a small pot over medium heat. Stir in the onion, celery, carrot, cook 5 minutes, until tender. Add chicken broth and heat through. Transfer to food processor, and puree until smooth. Return to pot and bring to boil. Stir in evaporated milk or half and half. Simmer 5 minutes. Season with salt and pepper.

Recipe Name: **Lentil Soup**
Portion Size: 1 ½ cup
Servings: 1 = 1 cup
Ingredients:
1 teaspoon olive oil
2 tablespoons carrots, washed, peeled and diced
2 tablespoons onion, chopped
2 tablespoons celery, chopped
1/3 cup lentils
¼ cup water
¼ teaspoon ground black pepper
1 tablespoon tomato paste
¼ teaspoon ground coriander
¼ teaspoon ground cumin
¼ teaspoon garlic powder
1/2 cup chicken broth
salt and pepper to taste.
Directions:

Wash and prepare vegetables. Heat the oil in a small pot over medium heat. Stir in the onion, celery, carrot, cook 5 minutes, until tender. Add chicken broth, water black pepper, coriander, cumin, garlic powder, and lentils. Bring to boil. Reduce heat to low. Simmer for 20 minutes until lentils are tender. Transfer to food processor, and puree until smooth. Return to pot and bring to boil. Stir in tomato paste. Simmer 5 minutes. Season with salt and pepper.

Recipe Name: **Cream of Potato Soup**

Portion Size: 1 cup
Servings: 1 = 1 cup
Ingredients:
1 teaspoon olive oil
1 large potato, washed, peeled and diced
2 tablespoons onion, chopped
2 tablespoons celery, chopped
½ teaspoon parsley flakes
¼ cup chicken broth
¼ cup evaporated milk or half and half
2 tablespoons shredded cheese
salt and pepper to taste.
Directions:

Wash and prepare vegetables. Heat the oil in a small pot over medium heat. Stir in the onion, celery, potatoes cook 5 minutes. Add chicken broth and cook until potato is tender. Transfer to food processor, and puree until smooth. Return to pot and bring to boil. Stir in evaporated milk or half and half and cheese. Simmer 5 minutes. Season with salt and pepper.

Recipe Name: **Spilt Pea** Soup
Portion Size: 1 ½ cup
Servings: 1 = 1 cup
Ingredients:
1 teaspoon olive oil
2 tablespoons carrots, washed, peeled and diced
2 tablespoons onion, chopped
2 tablespoons celery, chopped
1/3 cup dried spilt peas
½ cup water
¼ teaspoon garlic powder
1/2 cup chicken broth
salt and pepper to taste.
Directions:

Wash and prepare vegetables. Heat the oil in a small pot over medium heat. Stir in the onion, celery, carrot, cook 5 minutes, until tender. Add chicken broth, water, black pepper, garlic powder, and peas. Bring to boil. Reduce heat to low. Simmer for 20 minutes until peas are tender. Transfer to food processor, and puree until smooth. Return to pot and bring to boil. Simmer 5 minutes. Season with salt and pepper.

Recipe Name: **Tomato Basil Soup**
Portion Size: 1   cup
Servings: 1 = 1 cup
Ingredients:
1 teaspoon olive oil
2 tablespoons carrots, washed, peeled and diced
2 tablespoons celery, chopped
2 tablespoons onion, chopped
¼ teaspoon ground black pepper
¼ cup chicken broth
½ cup canned crushed tomatoes
2 tablespoons fresh basil, minced or 2 teaspoons dried basil
¼ cup evaporated milk or half and half
¼ teaspoon sugar
1 tablespoon Parmesan cheese
Directions:

Wash and prepare onions, and carrots. Heat the oil in a small pot over medium heat. Stir in the onion, celery, carrot, cook 5 minutes, until tender. Add chicken broth and heat through. Transfer to food processor, and puree until smooth. Return to pot and bring to boil. Stir in half and half or evaporated milk. Simmer 5 minutes. In a small bowl add 2 tablespoons soup to crushed tomatoes stir to temper. Add to soup with sugar and heat through.
Top with Parmesan cheese while hot.

Recipe Name: **White Bean Soup**
Portion Size: 1 1/4 cup
Servings: 1 = 1 cup
Ingredients:
1 tablespoon olive oil
2 tablespoons onion, chopped
1 small can (8oz.) white beans, drained and rinsed
2 tablespoons carrot, peeled and chopped
2 tablespoons celery
¼ cup chicken broth
1/4 teaspoon dried basil
salt and pepper to taste
¼ teaspoon dried thyme
¼ teaspoon dried parsley flakes

Directions:

Wash and prepare onions, celery, and carrots. Heat the oil in a small pot over medium heat. Stir in the onion, celery, and carrot. and cook 5 minutes, until tender. In a food processor, vegetables, beans, thyme, parsley, basil, and broth until smooth. Return to pot and bring to boil. Simmer 5 minutes. Season with salt and pepper.

Starch Side Dishes

Starches puree better when still hot. Puree spaghetti and other pastas separately and not with the accompanying sauce (i.e. spaghetti sauce, beef cubes). Puree plain rice is more difficult to process and can become very sticky. Substitute cream of rice seasoned with a complimentary sauce, gravy, or margarine. The sauce, gravy or margarine should be served as a topping for optimal flavor. Rice pilafs can be processed hot with a small amount of broth or milk.

Recipe Name: **Baked Acorn Squash**
(or can be made with other winter squashes like; Butternut Squash, Kabuki, Hubbard, Delicate, Blue Hokkaido, Pumpkin)
Portion Size: 1-2 cups
Servings: 1 = 1/2 cup
Ingredients:
1 Acorn squash, washed, halved and seeds removed.
1 tablespoon olive oil
2 tablespoons brown sugar
Salt and pepper to taste
¼ teaspoon ground cinnamon (optional)
Directions:

Preheat oven to 350 degrees. Place squash in a shallow baking pan, cut side down. Bake in preheated oven for 30 minutes. Turn cut side up; Season with salt and pepper, dot with olive oil and sprinkle with brown sugar and cinnamon. Bake for 20 minutes or until tender. Remove and peel squash in a food processor, combine all the ingredients. Blend until smooth.

Recipe Name: **Baked Beans**
Portion Size: 1 cup
Servings: 1 = ½ cup
Ingredients:
1 small can (8oz.) baked beans
½ teaspoon brown sugar
1 tablespoon ketchup
1 teaspoon prepared yellow mustard
¼ teaspoon Worcestershire sauce
2 tablespoons carrot, peeled and chopped

Directions:

Preheat oven to 350 degrees F. Combine all ingredients in a casserole dish. Bake 20 minutes or until hot and bubbly. This may also be made on the stove top. In a food processor, puree all ingredients. Blend until smooth

Recipe Name: **Black Beans**
Portion Size: 1 cup
Servings: 1 = 1 cup
Ingredients:
1 teaspoon olive oil
2 tablespoons onion, chopped
1 teaspoon dried cilantro flakes
1 small can (8oz.) black beans, drained and rinsed
2 tablespoons carrot, peeled and chopped
¼ teaspoon garlic powder
¼ teaspoon ground black pepper

Dash cayenne pepper (optional)

Directions:

Heat the oil in a small pot over medium heat. Stir in the onion, carrots, and cook 5 minutes, until tender. In a food processor onion, carrots, cilantro beans, cayenne pepper, and garlic powder puree until smooth. Return to pot and bring to boil. Simmer 5 minutes. Garnish with sour cream.

Recipe Name: **Mashed Potatoes**
Portion Size: 1   cup
Servings: 1 = ½ cup
Ingredients:
1 medium potato
1 tablespoon milk or cream
1 teaspoon butter or margarine
Salt and pepper to taste.
Optional: may add for variation. Add to food processor.
¼ teaspoon garlic powder or
2 tablespoons shredded cheese or
¼ teaspoon paprika or
¼ teaspoon of your favorite ground seasoning.

Directions:

Wash and peel potatoes. Cut into small pieces. Place in small pan. Cover with water. Cover and bring to a boil. Cook until tender. Drain. In a food processor, puree with milk and margarine or butter until smooth. Season with salt or pepper.

Vegetables

Vegetables come from various edible parts of plants. Vegetables come from the roots of plants, leaves of plants, stems of plants or flowers of plants.
Examples:
Roots: Beets, Carrots, Jicama, Parsnip, Radish, Rutabagas, Sweet Potatoes, Turnips
Tubers: Ginger root, Potatoes, Sun choke
Leaves: Beet greens, Bok Choy, Brussels Sprouts, Cabbage, Chard, Chinese Cabbage, Collard greens, Dandelion greens, Parsley, Romaine, Spinach, Turnip greens, Watercress
Stems and Shoots: Fennel, Asparagus, Celery, Kohlrabi
Flowers: Artichokes, Broccoli, Cauliflower
Seeds: Beans, Corn, Lentils, Peas

Vegetables are an excellent source of fiber. Processing vegetables does not decrease the fiber content. In fact, it can make them more bioavailable and may increase the body's ability to utilize the fiber. Fibers in vegetables are indigestible by human but can provide numerous health benefits. Two fibers in vegetables (and fruits) in are pectin and hemicellulose. The hemicellulose gives the plant structure in the cell walls of the plant. The outer layer of the skin, peel, and rind have a higher proportion and can make processing vegetables more difficult. Adding heat or an acid may help to break down these fibers and make processing easier. For example, for fresh spinach, cooking the spinach or adding a vingarette salad dressing will make processing easier.

Vegetables can add color and visual appeal to a plate. Vegetables (and fruits) have pigments and these pigments have positive health benefits. Cooking methods should be used to preserve nutrients and maintain color. Heat affects the color of vegetables because it modifies the structure of the pigments. Over heating or cooking vegetables should be avoided. Chlorophyll is the green pigment found in vegetables. To preserve the green color, vegetables can be blanched. To blanch vegetables, briefly dip the vegetables into boiling water. After blanching the vegetable, transfer the vegetables into an ice bath. Frozen vegetables may have already been blanched to preserve the color. Color changes in green vegetables can be minimized by keeping heat times short, adding small amounts of sugar and heating the food uncovered for the first few minutes. Avoid heating vegetables in a pan with a lid, or the pigment will change from bright green to dull green. To preserve the red-purple pigment of red cabbage or eggplant, adding an acid such as apple, lemon juice or vinegar. The white color of cauliflower, white potatoes, turnips or onions can be enhancing by adding an acid such as vinegar or lemon juice. For fresh beets, leave on 1-2 inches of the stem and peel the beets after cooking to prevent the rich red color from leaching into the water.

Make the vinaigrette by combining the cider vinegar, sugar, olive oil, and dry mustard.

To preserve nutrients and plant pigments, use only a minimal amount of liquid and a short cooking time. Vegetables should not be boiled, but instead simmered or steamed in as little water as possible.

The amount of carbohydrate and water vary by vegetables. Vegetables with a high starch content such as sweet potatoes, beans, peas, and potatoes tend to process very well and do not need very much liquid added (if any) when processed. Other vegetables with a higher water content will turn watery when process and will need a thickener to process. High water content vegetables include: cucumbers, tomatoes, and some lettuces. To provide nutrient dense vegetables, process first and only add liquid if necessary. If necessary apple or other 100% fruit juices can be added.

For green lettuce salads, choose arugula, romaine, Swiss chard, spinach, kale or any leafy green. Wash thoroughly and remove any tough stems or stalks. If necessary to get a smooth consistency add 1 teaspoon salad dressing per 1 cup serving greens. Top dressing on greens before serving. Greens should be served immediately after processing. If greens are too runny, thicken to consistency with instant potato flakes.

Vegetables

Recipe Name: **Steamed Vegetables**
Portion Size: 1/2 cup
Servings: 1 = ½ cup
Ingredients:
1 cup fresh or frozen vegetables of choice: Asparagus, Beets, Bell Peppers, Bok Choy, Broccoli, Brussels Sprouts, Cabbage, Carrots Cauliflower, Celery, Eggplant, Green Beans, Kale, Kohlrabi, Lima Beans, Mushrooms, Onions, Parsnips, Peas, Pea Pods, Spinach, Summer Squash, Wax Beans, Zucchini
1 teaspoon water
Directions:

Washed and prepare vegetables. Remove tough skins, seeds or fibrous stems. Place vegetables and water in a casserole dish and cover. Cook 2 to 10 minutes on high heat in microwave until vegetable are tender-crisp. Drain excess liquid. In a food processor, puree vegetable. Blend until smooth. Add thicken agent if too thin or runny. Vegetables should be the consistency of mashed potatoes. Serve.

Recipe Name: **Roasted** **Vegetables**
Portion Size: 1/2 cup
Servings: 1 = ½ cup
Ingredients:
1 cup fresh or frozen vegetables of choice Vegetables that roast well include: Asparagus, Beets, Broccoli, Brussels Sprouts, Cabbage, Carrots, Cauliflower, Celery, Green Beans, Eggplant, Kohlrabi, Mushrooms, Bell Peppers, Onions, Summer Squash, Tomatoes, Turnips and Winter Squash, Zucchini. Washed, trimmed, peeled, seeds removed and diced.
1 teaspoon oil
1 teaspoon dried parsley
¼ teaspoon garlic powder
¼ teaspoon paprika

Directions:

Washed and prepare vegetables. Remove tough skins, seeds or fibrous stems. Cut into uniform bite size pieces. Place on cookie sheet. Add olive oil, parsley, garlic and paprika. Toss to coat. Roast for 20 – 40 minutes, tossing occasionally until the vegetables are tender. In a food processor, puree vegetable. Blend until smooth. Add thicken agent if too thin or runny. Vegetables should be the consistency of mashed potatoes. Serve.

Vegetable Salads

Recipe Name: **Pickled Beets**
Portion Size: 1   cup
Servings: 1 = ½ cup
Ingredients:
1 (8 oz.) can diced beets, drained
1 teaspoon cider vinegar
1/4 teaspoon sugar
1 teaspoon olive oil
dash dry mustard
¼ teaspoon salt
¼ teaspoon pepper
Directions:

Make the vinaigrette by combining the cider vinegar, sugar, olive oil, salt, pepper and dry mustard. In a food processor, add beets. Blend until smooth. Add thickening agent if too thin. Place beets in serving dish. Top with dressing. Serve immediately, or refrigerate in a covered container.

Recipe Name: **Broccoli Salad**
This can also be made with other vegetables like beets, carrots, green beans, cauliflower or zucchini.
Portion Size: 1/2 cup
Servings: 1 = ½ cup
Ingredients:
1 cup fresh or frozen broccoli
1 tablespoon sour cream
1 tablespoon mayonnaise
¼ teaspoon lemon juice
Dash of salt and pepper
Directions:

Make the dressing by combining the mayonnaise, sour cream, salt, pepper and lemon juice. Steam broccoli in microwave with ½ teaspoon water. In a food processor, add broccoli. Blend until smooth. Add thickening agent if too thin. Place broccoli in serving dish. Top with dressing. Serve immediately, or refrigerate in a covered container.

Vegetables Smoothies

Vegetables smoothies are a great way to get vegetable servings. Adding vegetables to fruit smoothies is a tasty way to incorporate more vegetables.

Recipe Name: **Carrot Mango Smoothie**
Portion Size: 1 1/2 cups
Servings: 1 ½ cup
Ingredients:
2 large carrots, washed, trimmed, peeled and sliced
1 cup fresh or frozen mango, washed, peeled, seed removed and cut into small pieces
1 banana, peeled and sliced
1 teaspoon honey (optional)
1 red, yellow or orange bell pepper, trimmed and seeds removed.
Directions:
Thoroughly wash all produce. Pierce sweet potato with a few holes with a fork. Place carrots and peppers with 1 teaspoon water in microwave safe dish. Cover and microwave on high for 3--5 minutes on high or until tender. Let cool. In a food processor, combine all the ingredients. Blend until smooth. Chill.

Recipe Name: **Kale Lime Smoothie**
Portion Size: 1 1/2 cups
Servings: 1 ½ cup
Ingredients:
1 banana
½ cup fresh kale, stems removed
1 fresh lime juiced and zest
1 tablespoon honey or more to taste
Directions:
Thoroughly wash all vegetables and fruits. Prepare produce by washing, peeling, trimming and removing seeds or tough fibers. In a food processor, combine all the ingredients. Blend until smooth.

Recipe Name: **Mango Kale Smoothie**
Portion Size: 1 1/2 cups
Servings: 1 ½ cup
Ingredients:
1 cup frozen or fresh mango
½ cup fresh kale, stems removed
¼ cup white grape juice
Directions:
Thoroughly wash all vegetables and fruits. Prepare produce by washing, peeling, trimming and removing seeds or tough fibers. In a food processor, combine all the ingredients. Blend until smooth.

Recipe Name: **Pumpkin Spice Smoothie**
Portion Size: 1 1/2 cups
Servings: 1 ½ cup
Ingredients:
1 cup canned pumpkin puree
1 banana, peeled and cut into slices
¼ cup milk
1 teaspoon ground cinnamon or pumpkin spice
¼ teaspoon vanilla extract
1 tablespoon whipped topping (optional)
Directions:
Thoroughly wash sweet potato. Pierce sweet potato with a few holes with a fork. Place in microwave safe dish. Microwave on high for 5-7 minutes on high or until tender. Let cool. Peel. In a food processor, combine all the ingredients. Blend until smooth.

Recipe Name: **Spring Green Smoothie**
Portion Size: 1 1/2 cups
Servings: 1 ½ cup
Ingredients:
½ cup fresh asparagus, trimmed and cut into 1 inch pieces
¾ cup fresh baby spinach, stems removed
¼ cup white grape juice
1 ripe green apple or pear, peeled, seeds removed and coarsely chopped
Directions:
Thoroughly wash all vegetables and fruits. Prepare produce by washing, peeling, trimming and removing seeds or tough fibers. In a food processor, combine all the ingredients. Blend until smooth.

Recipe Name: **Spinach Ginger Smoothie**
Portion Size: 1 1/2 cups
Servings: 1 ½ cup
Ingredients:
2 cups fresh spinach, trimmed
1 ripe sliced banana
½ cup plain or vanilla nonfat yogurt
1 small apple, washed, peeled, seeds and core removed
¼ teaspoon ginger
1 lime juiced
Directions:
Thoroughly wash all vegetables and fruits. Prepare produce by washing, peeling, trimming and removing seeds or tough fibers. In a food processor, combine all the ingredients. Blend until smooth.

Recipe Name: **Spinach Kale Smoothie**
Portion Size: 1 1/2 cups
Servings: 1 ½ cup
Ingredients:
2 cups fresh spinach, trimmed
1/2 cup fresh kale, stems removed
1 tablespoon peanut butter
1 ripe sliced banana
½ cup plain or vanilla nonfat yogurt
Directions:
Thoroughly wash all vegetables and fruits. Prepare produce by washing, peeling, trimming and removing seeds or tough fibers. In a food processor, combine all the ingredients. Blend until smooth.

Recipe Name: **Spinach Peanut Butter Smoothie**
Portion Size: 1 1/2 cups
Servings: 1 ½ cup
Ingredients:
1/2 cup fresh spinach, stems removed
1 cup plain Greek yogurt
1 banana
3 ice cubes (optional)
Directions:
Thoroughly wash all vegetables and fruits. Prepare produce by washing, peeling, trimming and tough fibers. In a food processor, combine all the ingredients. Blend until smooth.

Recipe Name: **Sweet Potato Spice Smoothie**
Portion Size: 1 1/2 cups
Servings: 1 ½ cup
Ingredients:
1 large sweet potato
1 banana, peeled and cut into slices
¼ cup milk
1 teaspoon ground cinnamon or pumpkin spice
Directions:
Thoroughly wash sweet potato. Pierce sweet potato with a few holes with a fork. Place in microwave safe dish. Microwave on high for 5-7 minutes on high or until tender. Let cool. Peel. In a food processor, combine all the ingredients. Blend until smooth.

Recipe Index

Beverages:
Banana Berry Fruit Smoothie 49
Berry Pineapple Fruit Smoothie 49
Chocolate Banana Smoothie 50
Fruited Yogurt Drink 50
High Protein Milk 50
Mango Banana Smoothie 51
Raspberry Peach Smoothie 51
Orange Breakfast Sipper 51
Orange Frosty 52
Papaya Strawberry Smoothie 52
Peanut Butter Banana Smoothie 52
Pina Colada Smoothie 53
Pineapple Banana Sipper 53
Pudding Milkshakes 53
Pumpkin Banana Smoothie 54
Raspberry Banana Smoothie 54
High Calorie High Protein Shakes 54
Tofu Fruit Smoothie 55

Breads
Banana Bread in a Mug 56
Pumpkin Bread in a Mug 57
Pear Bread in a Mug 58
Apple Bread in a Mug 59

Desserts
Brownie in a Mug 60
Chocolate Cake in a Mug 61
Lemon Cake in a Mug 62
Peanut Butter Cookie in a Mug 63
Vanilla Cake in a Mug 64

Dinner Entrees
Beef
Asian Skirt Steak 67
Ground Beef Patty 68
Mini Meatloaf 69
Salisbury Steak 70

Chicken
Apple Spiced Chicken 71
Sauté Chicken 72
Chicken with Curry Sauce 73
Chicken Schnitzel 73
Chicken with Apple Mustard Sauce (or Pork) 74
Chicken with Apricot Ginger Teriyaki Sauce (or Pork) 76
Chicken with Dijon Sauce (or Pork) 77
Chicken with Cacciatore Sauce 78
Chicken with Curry Mango Sauce (or Pork) 79
Chicken with Honey Orange Sauce (or Pork) 80
Chicken with Orange Mustard Sauce (or Pork) 81
Chicken with Lemon Sauce 82
Chicken with Spiced Peach Sauce (or Pork) 83
Italian Chicken 84
Sesame Ginger Chicken 85

Pork
Pork Chop with Chili Rub 86
Pork Chop with Cranberry Apple Sauce (or chicken) 87
Pork Chop with Apple Curry Sauce (or chicken) 88
Pork Chop with Fresh Plum Sauce (or chicken) 89
Pork Chop with Honey Garlic Sauce (or chicken) 90
Pork Chops with Sour Cream Sauce (or chicken) 91

Seafood
Baked Cod with Lemon Dill Sauce 92
Blacken Tilapia Fish 93
Broiled Parmesan Fish 94
Crab Cakes & Red Pepper Sauce 95
Glazed Salmon 96
Lemon Dijon Baked Fish 97
Salmon Patties with Cheese Sauce (or Tuna or Crab) 81
Shrimp with Marinated Chili Garlic Sauce 99
Tuna Cakes with Creamy Citrus Sauce 100

Dinner Turkey
Cranberry Turkey Steaks 101
Ground Turkey Patty (beef or chicken) 102
Tarragon Turkey Patty (or chicken) 103
Spicy Turkey Meatballs 104
Ground Turkey with Mushroom Sauce 105

Salad Dressing
Asian Ginger Dressing 107
Avocado Cilantro Dressing 107
Balsamic Honey Mustard Dressing 108
Basil and Garlic Vinaigrette Dressing 108
Blue Cheese Dressing 109
Buttermilk Dressing 109
Carrot Ginger Dressing 110
Citrus Dressing 110
Citrus Parmesan Dressing 111
Creamy Basil Dressing 111
Creamy Italian Dressing 112
Creamy Lemon Garlic Salad Dressing 112
Lemon Dijon Vinaigrette 113
Dill Dressing 113
French Dressing 114
Greek Dressing 114
Honey Mustard Dressing 115
Ranch Buttermilk Dressing 115
Southwestern Salad Dressing 116
Sweet and Sour Oriental Dressing 116
Sweet Dijon Mustard Dressing 116
Tangy Basil Vinaigrette Dressing 117
Tangy Lime Dressing 117
Thousand Island Dressing 118

Sauces
Aioli Garlic Sauce 119
Alfredo Sauce 119
Apple Yogurt Sauce 120
Basil Aioli Sauce 120
Basil Sauce 121
Blueberry Sauce (or other fruit) 121
Chili Garlic Sauce 122
Chipotle Sauce 122
Cilantro Avocado Sauce 122
Cranberry Mustard Sauce 123
Creamy Cantaloupe Sauce 123
Creamy Dill Sauce 123
Creamy Paprika Sauce 124
Creamy Parmesan Garlic Sauce 124
Creamy Tomato Basil Sauce 125
Curry Sauce 126
Feta Yogurt Sauce 126
Garlic Curry Sauce 127
Honey Mustard Sauce 128
Hot Fudge Sauce 128
Lemon Dill Yogurt Sauce 128
Marinara Sauce 129
Mexican Sauce 130
Mushroom Sauce 130
Orange Dipping Sauce 130
Pan Gravy 131
Peach Ginger Sauce 131

Peanut Sauce 132
Pesto Sauce 132
Plum Sauce 133
Seafood Sauce 133
Spicy Mango Sauce 134
Tahini Yogurt Sauce 134
Tartar Sauce 135
Teriyaki Sauce 135

Soups
Baked Acorn Squash Soup (or Butternut) 136
Black Bean Soup 137
Black Eyed Pea Chowder 138
Carrot Ginger Soup 138
Cream of Carrot Soup (or Vegetable) 139
Lentil Soup 140
Cream of Potato Soup 141
Spilt Pea Soup 142
Tomato Basil Bisque 143
White Bean Soup 144

Starchy Side Dish
Baked Acorn Squash 145
Baked Beans 146
Black Beans 146
Mashed Potatoes 147

Vegetable
Steamed Vegetables 151
Roasted Vegetables 152

Vegetable Salads
Pickled Beets 153
Broccoli Salad (or another veg.) 154

Vegetable Smoothies
Carrot Mango Smoothie 155
Kale Lime Smoothie 156
Mango Kale Smoothie 156
Pumpkin Spice Smoothie 157
Spring Green Smoothie 157
Spinach Ginger Smoothie 158
Spinach Kale Smoothie 158
Spinach Peanut Butter Smoothie 159
Sweet Potato Spice Smoothie 159

www.ingramcontent.com/pod-product-compliance
Lightning Source LLC
Chambersburg PA
CBHW081149180526
45170CB00006B/1988